ANIMALS AND MEDICINE

Animals and Medicine

The Contribution of Animal Experiments to the Control of Disease

Jack H. Botting
edited by Regina M. Botting

OpenBook Publishers

http://www.openbookpublishers.com

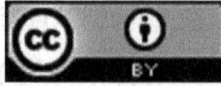

Digital material and resources associated with this volume are available at http://www.openbookpublishers.com/isbn/9781783741175#resources

ISBN Paperback: 978-1-78374-117-5
ISBN Hardback: 978-1-78374-118-2
ISBN Digital (PDF): 978-1-78374-119-9
ISBN Digital ebook (epub): 978-1-78374-120-5
ISBN Digital ebook (mobi): 978-1-78374-121-2
DOI: 10.11647/OBP.0055

Cover image: Pancreas and insulin (image B0007641). Wellcome Library, London, CC BY.

All paper used by Open Book Publishers is SFI (Sustainable Forestry Initiative), and PEFC (Programme for the Endorsement of Forest Certification Schemes) Certified.

Printed in the United Kingdom and United States by Lightning Source for Open Book Publishers

Contents

III. Drugs for Organic Diseases

List of Illustrations

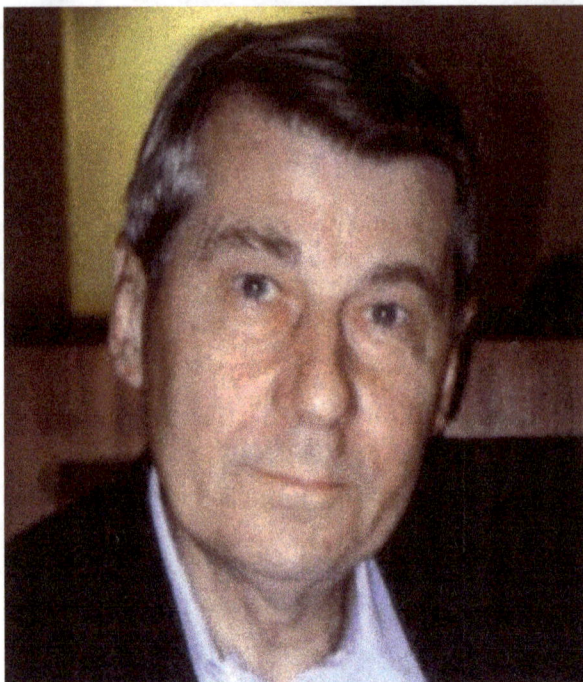

Dr. J.H. Botting, 6 January 1932-12 July 2012

Jack Howard Botting was born in Croydon, London and attended Selhurst Grammar School where he developed his lifelong passion for Rugby and captained the School First Fifteen. He graduated B.Pharm at Chelsea College in 1954 and immediately commenced postgraduate research under the supervision of Professor Mary Lockett.

On completing his Ph.D. in 1957, Jack entered National Service in the Royal Army Medical Corps and was posted to Army Operational Research Group. Seconded to the MRC Laboratories at Holly Hill, London he carried out research on acclimatization to heat and the assessment of stress in human subjects. In 1959 Jack returned to Chelsea as Lecturer in Pharmacology at a time when pharmacology was entering a golden age of drug research and discovery. Chelsea had many fine and dedicated teachers but Jack was exceptional in his eye for detail and in the pastoral care of his students. Liaison with industrial and government research centres was an important part of his responsibilities which allowed him to secure places for students in their third year intercalated research course. Many former students have spoken warmly of how Jack helped them obtain positions after graduating and how he would keep track of their careers.

Jack himself had a year's sabbatical at the Sandoz Laboratories in Basel (1969-70) and returned as Senior Lecturer to Chelsea until 1989 when he became acting Head of Department prior and during the merger of Kings and Chelsea College. In 1990 he decided to retire from academic life and took the position of Scientific Director of the Research Defence Society until he finally retired in 1995.

Jack held many influential positions on academic committees in the University of London (as it was) including the chairmanship of the Board of Studies in Pharmacology. His major contributions to teaching pharmacology was recognised by the Society by the award of the Rang Prize in 2011.

Jack married Renia Botting, a fellow Chelsea student, in 1958 and Renia was still at his side when he left us in July 2012.

Foreword

Animals and Medicine: The Contribution of Animal Experiments to the Control of Disease presents a detailed, scholarly historical review of the critical role experiments using animals have played in advancing medical knowledge. Laboratory animals have been essential, and the knowledge gained has saved countless human lives – and not only human lives. Animals, themselves, have benefitted. Unfortunately, those opposed to using animals in research, some even physicians, have presented doctored evidence that using animals has impeded medical progress. Therefore, the articles Jack Botting wrote for the *Research Defence Society News* from 1991 to 1996 have provided scientists – those willing to speak out – with the information needed to rebut such foolish claims.

Of course, animals are only used when necessary and other methods will not answer the question posed. It must be admitted that in days gone by attention to their welfare was not uppermost in the minds of some scientists. In the modern era, though, laboratory animal medicine has made major advances, and scientists are enjoined legally and morally to follow the principles of the 3Rs expounded by Russell and Burch: reduction (in numbers used); refinement (of experimental techniques to eliminate or reduce pain); and replacement (with alternative approaches when available).[1] An extensive philosophical defence of the use of animals can be found elsewhere.[2]

It is tragic that Jack's book had to be published posthumously. But thankfully, his efforts to put his many articles into book form were not initiated in vain because his wife, Regina, has carried his work on to publication.

---

1   Russell W M S and Burch (1959), *The Principles of Humane Experimental Technique*. London: Metheun.
2   Morrison A R (2009), *An Odyssey with Animals: Reflections of a Veterinarian on the Animal Rights & Welfare Debate*. Oxford: Oxford University Press.

http://dx.doi.org/10.11647/OBP.0055.20

Because Jack and I had collaborated on a few articles more than fifteen years ago, she asked me if I would introduce the book.

Ours was a curious collaboration because we never had the pleasure of meeting face-to-face. But on the basis of one telephone call and numerous emails we wrote three essays. The first was written for an ill-conceived debate organized by *Scientific American*. Jack had been invited by the magazine to write an article defending the need for using animals in biomedical research.[3] Jack thought that it would be best to have an American join him in the debate and chose me because I had been very active in the field.

Our opponents were to be two physicians, Neal Barnard and Stephen Kaufman, well-known for philosophical objection to using animals and their false claims that animal research has been wasteful and misleading. We knew that they had a history of depending on gross and clever distortions of medical history to support those claims, and what they wrote for the debate was no exception.[4] Having joined together, Jack and I then tried to persuade the editor that his debate would be unwise and harmful because, as planned, there would be no chance for rebuttal. Our plea fell on deaf ears even after we had seen the contributions of our opponents prior to publication and had pointed out to the editor their various distortions of history requiring a reply.

The editor's answer was that the issue was an important one and should be presented to the public as planned. But how was an uninformed public to sort out fact from fancy, we asked? Barnard and Kaufman's philosophical objections to using animals in research had been melded into a supposedly scientifically sound presentation of medical history.

Regrettably, the debate was published; and, as we had predicted, reference to Barnard's and Kaufman's article in what had always been a legitimate journal began to appear in animal-rightist publications. Although one scientist whose work had been misrepresented wrote a letter to the editor describing how his statements had been presented wrongly, Jack and I thought that an extensive rebuttal had to be published somewhere. We found two outlets for presenting our rebuttal: an online journal, *H.M.S. Beagle: TheBioMedNet*

---

3   Botting J H and Morrison A R (1997), Animal research is vital to medicine. *Sci Am* 276 (2) 83-85.

4   Barnard N D and Kaufman S R Animal research is wasteful and misleading, *Sci Am* 276 (2) 80-82. http://dx.doi.org/10.1038/scientificamerican0297-80

magazine,[5] and a guest editorial in *The American Biology Teacher*.[6] The former is defunct, but science and medical journalist, Andrew A. Skolnick, is kindly hosting the article on his website.

We actually based our article in HMS Beagle, 'UnScientific American: Animal Rights or Wrongs,' on the several emails we had sent to the editor of *Scientific American* detailing Barnard's and Kaufman's distortions of medical history on several fronts. Our corrections focused on the development of the polio vaccine, stroke research, drug side effects, the birth defects induced by thalidomide, and the miracle of insulin. These topics are among the many that are discussed in this book in incredible detail.

Our guest editorial, 'Confusion in the Ranks' allowed us to present our arguments to an extremely important audience: biology teachers. Animalrightist propaganda had been infecting young minds for many years so we thought it critical to counter these efforts. The misleading methods presented in *Scientific American* and elsewhere were listed

in no particular order of perversity [as we put it]:

1. Overemphasizing an ultimate clinical discovery while ignoring the dependence on years of dedicated background laboratory work of others or else dismissing the need to dissect mechanisms after a clinical observation
2. Endowing a particular methodology, such as epidemiology, with exaggerated powers
3. Reporting experimental observations or even the opinions of scientists out of context
4. Using faulty logic
5. Reversing the conclusions of a particular article by quoting a disjointed series of sentences as if they had appeared together in the original
6. Boldly listing supporting references even if they are not. (6, p. 388)

We then offered something positive: ideas for creating a curriculum module around the debate. First among them was the philosophical question of whether we are justified in using animals for purposes of our own health

5 Botting J H and Morrison A R (1998) UnScientific American: animal rights or wrongs: An op-ed. *HMS Beagle: TheBioMedNetMagazine* 25 (Feb 20) 1-7, http://www.aaskolnick.com/morrison/unscian.htm

6 Morrison A R and Botting J H (1997), Confusion in the ranks *Am Biol Teacher* 59 388-89. http://dx.doi.org/10.2307/4450341

and well-being. If the answer is negative, is the individual prepared to live without benefitting from medical advances? We then suggested asking students how one would develop new drugs or surgical techniques without using animals in one or more stages of the process. Finally, we suggested researching one of the claims made in the *Scientific American* debate. We noted that the editor had received references from both sets of authors so that the magazine should be able to provide them on request. I hope some did follow through on this last suggestion. The foregoing illustrates how important Jack's efforts were. I hope that many scientists will make good use of them in public education.

Adrian R. Morrison, DVM, PhD
Professor Emeritus of Behavioral Neuroscience
School of Veterinary Medicine, University of Pennsylvania
Philadelphia, PA, USA

Introduction

The Research Defence Society (RDS) was founded in 1908 by Dr Stephen Paget, son of the eminent Victorian surgeon, Sir James Paget. Its role was to defend scientists conducting medical research using animals and to inform the public about the importance of animal experimentation. In its first year it attracted a membership of 2000 which included scientists in the pharmaceutical industry, in academia and in research institutes. Past presidents of the Society include such distinguished figures as Lord Perry of Walton and Sir William Paton.

Dr Jack Botting joined the staff of the RDS as its Scientific Officer in 1991, at the height of the antivivisectionist activity being carried out by organisations such as the Animal Liberation Front (ALF), the National Anti-Vivisection Society (NAVS), the British Union for the Abolition of Vivisection (BUAV) and People for the Ethical Treatment of Animals (PETA).

One of the most damaging aspects of antivivisection campaigning was that they had started to hijack the scientific argument, claiming that animal experimentation was scientifically misleading, "a failed technology" etc., and that an examination of the research behind major medical advances showed that non-animal techniques were crucial and that the animal experiments had contributed nothing, or worse still, held up progress. Antivivisectionists were deliberately shifting the debate from the traditional "science vs animal welfare" argument to a "scientific" debate giving their arguments a cover of scientific respectability.

To respond to this style of campaigning, Jack was given the specific task of reviewing the research behind the major medical advances and writing non-technical reviews explaining the role played by animal experimentation. His work effectively put an end to this aspect of antivivisection campaigning. The articles which Jack wrote at that time have been collected in this book.

But the activists didn't stop at spreading misinformation. Some extremist groups harassed, threatened and attacked scientists and laboratories involved

http://dx.doi.org/10.11647/OBP.0055.21

in animal research, painting graffiti on the houses of researchers and even planting bombs under their cars. Colin Blakemore, Professor of Physiology at Oxford University, who was recognised for his research in early 2014 with a knighthood, was one of those targeted by these groups. A leading vision scientist who has used cats for his studies, he has received letter bombs, death threats against him and his family, had his car damaged and the windows of his home broken. The activists also agitated to close down laboratories which used animals and the facilities which bred them. Meanwhile, scientists were working to find ways to refine and reduce the use of animals in research, but their efforts did not appease the antivivisectionists who were determined to shut down animal research altogether.

These antivivisectionist groups vary in size and structure; PETA, for example, claims that their membership runs into millions. This particular group has a wide campaign portfolio: as well as vivisection, it also protests against the use of animals for fur farming, pet ownership, hunting and even for food. They and groups like them receive large donations from which they obtain a considerable income – PETA receives millions of pounds annually from their supporters.

The current animal rights movement, with its organised activities, has its origins in the publication of the book *Animal Liberation* in 1975, by Australian philosopher Peter Singer, which animal liberationists viewed as providing their founding philosophical statement of ideas. The following year saw the foundation of the ALF, followed in the 1980s by the Animal Rights Militia, which, as its name suggests, was an extreme group which sent bombs to politicians and animal researchers. In the early 1990s, they and other similar groups firebombed scientists and organisations engaged in medical research using animals.

One of the most well-known activists is Greg Avery, who founded Stop Huntingdon Animal Cruelty (SHAC) in 1999 and is an alleged member of the ALF. He was involved with a 10-month campaign that succeeded in closing down Consort Kennels, a facility which bred beagles for medical research. From 1996, Avery was in and out of prison on various charges before being jailed for nine years in 2008 after being convicted of conspiracy to blackmail; imprisoned along with him were his wife and ex-wife. Other protests achieved some success: 1999 saw the closure of Hillgrove Cat Farm, the last dedicated UK establishment which bred cats, its owner retiring after a sustained series of protests and attacks. In 2005 the Hall brothers, owners of Newchurch Guinea Pig Farm, shut up shop after a six-year campaign by activists; in one two-year period police logged 450 separate criminal acts.

The victimisation culminated in the theft of the remains of Christopher Hall's mother-in-law and, although no one was ever convicted of the desecration of the grave, four people were jailed for using the theft to blackmail the family.[1]

The degree of criminal behaviour exhibited by these groups led the British government to set up the National Extremism Tactical Coordination Unit (NETCU) which aimed to enable the police to deal effectively with animal rights extremism. In addition, legislation has been put in place to curb the activity of antivivisection groups. These measures, combined with more severe sentences handed down by judges, have notably reduced extremist action by such groups.

At the same time, the press coverage given to the more extreme cases led to public condemnation of the tactics animal liberation groups were using and along with this came an increase in awareness of the issues involved. While new animal rights campaigns were set up, other groups were formed, such as Speaking of Research, to counter them. In 2003, the work of the RDS was reinforced by the establishment of the Coalition for Medical Progress (CMP), which also engaged in pro-research communication. At the end of 2008, the two organisations merged to form Understanding Animal Research (UAR). The announcement of the building of a new animal research facility, the Oxford Biomedical Research Institute, resulted in animal rights extremists burning down student boathouses at Oxford University in protest. This action led to the formation at the beginning of 2006 of the Pro-Test committee and in February of that year they held their first rally, which saw over 800 students, scientists and members of the public marching through Oxford in support of animal research. Two subsequent rallies again attracted hundreds of people and, in 2008, Oxford University opened its new Biomedical Sciences Building.[2]

This tide of public support has been complemented by the pursuit of alternatives to animal research by the scientific community. The charity, Fund for the Replacement of Animals in Medical Experiments (FRAME), was registered in 1969 and has provided a blueprint for similar organisations throughout Europe and in the USA, advising the government on the Animals (Scientific Procedures) Act, passed in 1986. Medical research was still being regulated by the 1876 Cruelty to Animals Act, which was in need of updating. FRAME outlined a 'Three Rs' approach, advocating the replacement, reduction and refinement of experiments on animals and the work of the organisation,

---

1 Illman J (2008) *Animal Research in Medicine: 100 Years of Politics, Protests and Progress. The Story of the Research Defence Society.* London: Research Defence Society.

2 Holder T (2014) 'Standing up for Science: The Antivivisection Movement and How to Stand up to It.' *EMBO Reports* 15/6, 625-30, http://dx.doi.org/10.1002/embr.201438837

along with progress in scientific knowledge, has enabled the first of these to become a reality. The LD50 test has been substituted by the ED50 test which uses fewer animals; the Pyrogen Test using live rabbits has been supplanted by the Limulus Amebocyte Lysate (LAL) Assay which uses the blood of the limulus crab, and the potency of a batch of insulin is now determined by biochemical methods instead of the blood sugar levels of conscious rabbits.

Animal rights extremism has been significantly curbed due to the measures mentioned above, as well as the restraining or imprisonment of many of the most zealous activists. 2014 finally saw the end of the campaign against Huntingdon Life Sciences (HLS). The sustained attacks on Huntingdon had seen not only staff targeted but also investors; they received hoax bombs, had their cars torched and one US executive even had his boat sunk. Much of the energy of the activists has now been channelled into online campaigns, with antivivisection groups campaigning to stop airlines transporting primates, having already successfully prevented ferry companies transporting laboratory animals across the English Channel.[3]

The debates around animal experimentation will continue and animal rights activists will continue to campaign. However, the landscape has changed considerably and there are several organisations now engaged in countering the campaigner's arguments and disseminating information. In the UK, the work of UAR is supported by the charitable organisation, the Biomedical Research Education Trust (BRET), which was originally set up by the RDS and which supports lectures for schools and societies interested in finding out the facts about animal research. In the USA, the groups Americans for Medical Progress (AMP) and the Foundation for Medical Research (FMR) perform a similar role. Even at the time of writing this introduction one of the recipients of the 2014 Nobel Prize for Physiology or Medicine, John O'Keefe, spoke in support of the use of animals. In an interview with the BBC he said "It is an incontrovertible fact that if we are to make progress in basic areas of medicine and biology, we are going to have to use animals."[4]

This volume of Jack's articles is supported by the trustees of BRET and their generosity is gratefully acknowledged. I would also like to thank Josephine Botting, Nina Botting Herbst and Mark Matfield for skilful editing and Ian O'Sullivan for invaluable technical help.

Regina Botting, Ph.D., October 2014

---

3   *The Independent on Sunday* (2014) Animal rights group ends campaign, 24th August 2014.

4   BBC News Website, Interview with John O'Keefe by James Gallagher, 7th October 2014.

I. TREATMENT OF INFECTIOUS DISEASES

1. Smallpox and After: An Early History of the Treatment and Prevention of Infections

The scientific work that led to the discovery of the causes of infections was possibly the major biomedical advance of the nineteenth century. From it was derived the aseptic technique of Lister, the use of antitoxins and immunisation, and the ultimately successful search for chemicals selectively toxic to bacterial cells.

The conquest of most of the infectious diseases is, however, the field subjected to the most derisive attack by the antivivisectionists. The scourges that were responsible for the high childhood mortality up to the end of the nineteenth century were, it is claimed, defeated by improvements in sanitation, nutrition and housing, rather than knowledge obtained from animal experimentation.

Improvements in public health undoubtedly contributed to the reduction in death from infectious disease. Obviously the easiest way to avoid morbidity is to stay away from the cause. However, with one notable exception, the causes are still with us. The tubercle bacillus, streptococcus, poliovirus etc. could still, even in our sanitary environment, cause lethal or crippling conditions if there was no appropriate medical intervention. The fact that 50 million prescriptions for antibiotics are written per year in the UK is testimony to the continued prevalence of infective disease.

Pasteur and others, in the second half of the nineteenth century, attributed the cause of certain diseases to microbes that enter (or infect) the body. Pasteur's subsequent work, on the examination of the relative virulence of microbes

http://dx.doi.org/10.11647/OBP.0055.01

after *in vitro* culture, put a sound scientific basis beneath the empirical practice of smallpox vaccination that was current in Europe at the time.

Smallpox

Those who may harbour in their imagination an affinity for the romanticism of pre-Victorian times would find the historical descriptions of smallpox sobering reading. De la Condamine (1) wrote in 1754:

> Every tenth death was due to smallpox, and one fourth of mankind were either killed by it, or crippled or disfigured for life. The disease was a river that everyone had to cross.

This severe scourge was endemic in China and other eastern countries centuries before Christ and was certainly present in Europe in the sixth century.

Bishop Gregory of Tours was surely describing smallpox when he wrote in 582 of the epidemic with vesicular eruption (*lues cum vesicis*) which began with sickness, fever and back pains. The fever abated with the copious eruption of hard, white vesicles which were very painful. Bad cases were fatal (amongst the young especially) on the 12th to 14th day.

The prevalence of the disease in these early times is indicated by the first clear description of smallpox by a physician. This was that of Isaacus Judaeus, or Isaac the Jew, who lived in the ninth century. Isaac theorised, since smallpox attacked everyone, that it was a natural fermentation of the blood in children in order to get rid of an impurity acquired in the womb. That smallpox continued to be a widespread scourge up to the time of the formal record of morbidity and mortality is evidenced by the quotation of De la Condamine (see above).

Against this background it is not hard to understand the development of the technique of inoculation (or variolation). This was the deliberate infection of pustular matter, collected during a mild epidemic, into an incision in a healthy child. This practice stemmed from the clinical observation that one attack of smallpox conferred protection against the disease and was long used by physicians of ancient China and India. It was introduced into Europe in 1721 by Lady Mary Wortley Montague, wife of the British Ambassador to Turkey. Although efficacious, the procedure was extremely dangerous, causing at least three epidemics on the continent and being fatal in at least 1-2% of cases (2). That individuals were prepared to accept discomfort and such severe risks attests to the inevitability with which people accepted smallpox in the era before any statistics were available.

Vaccination

Jenner's experiments, published in 1798, obviated the need for variolation and set the scene for the eventual eradication of smallpox. The story is familiar. Jenner, like others before, was intrigued by the accepted belief that individuals who came into contact with the comparatively rare disease of cowpox were immune to smallpox. In his classic experiment Jenner inoculated a boy with pus from a cowpox lesion on the hand of an infected dairymaid. Two months later the boy was inoculated with pus from a smallpox vesicle but did not develop the disease. "Vaccination" with cowpox resulted in immunity to smallpox. Vaccination gradually spread throughout Europe during the next hundred years.

The Vaccine

Initially vaccination was usually effected by the use of "humanised" lymph that is a lymph from the pustules of those previously vaccinated. The occasional accidental transmission of syphilis and the lack of sufficient vaccine material to combat an epidemic led to the use of animals to prepare the vaccine. Horses, mules, goats and rabbits were all used at one time to generate the virus. However calves became the standard method to prepare the vaccine, due to the facility with which the supply could be multiplied at relatively short notice to deal with even the most serious epidemic. The potency of the prepared virus was tested by the rapidity with which it could produce lesions in rabbits (3), it was usually also tested on mice to ensure the absence of tetanus bacilli (3).

The Effects of Vaccination

Where the introduction of vaccination was extended the immediate result was "a striking and rapid fall of smallpox mortality" (2). Fortunately the recording of local or national morbidity and mortality statistics became common at this time and thus the beneficial effect of vaccination was immediately apparent.

Sweden

Sweden was one of the earliest countries to vaccinate extensively. Vaccination began in Lund in 1801 and 25,000 were so treated by 1805. From 1805 on about 20,000 vaccinations per year were performed. Vaccination was made compulsory in 1816. The effect was dramatic. Average annual deaths per million population during the decades 1792-1801, 1802-11 and 1812-21 were 1,914, 623 and 133 respectively (Fig. 1.1).

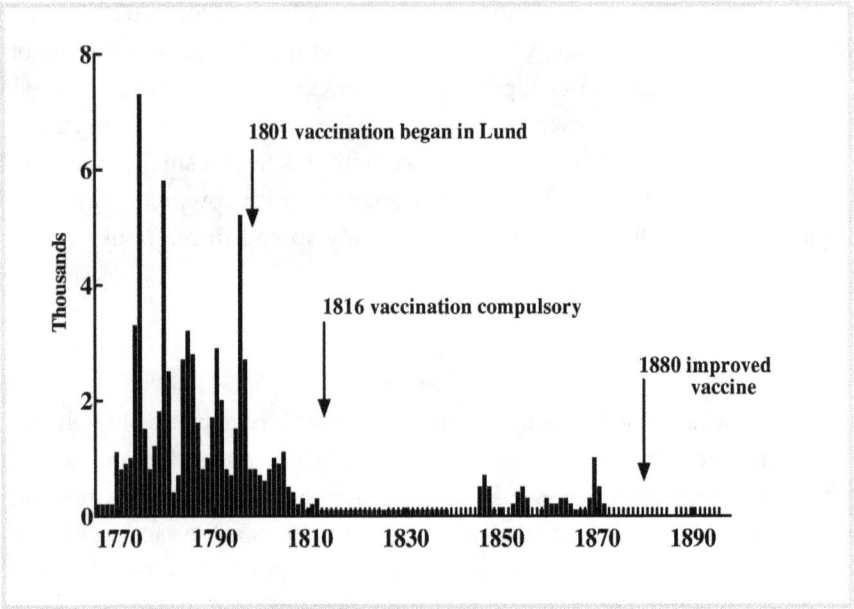

Fig. 1.1 Smallpox deaths in Sweden, 1774-1900.

Bavaria

Bavaria, in 1807, was the first country to make vaccination compulsory. Smallpox deaths were reduced and the disease became more prevalent in older persons rather than children. This pointed to the necessity for revaccination, which was made compulsory in 1872, after which smallpox virtually died out in that country.

Netherlands

The Netherlands adopted compulsory vaccination in 1873 and an attenuation in smallpox mortality was immediately apparent.

England

In England vaccination was made obligatory in infancy in 1853 and compulsory under punishment in 1867, although it is alleged that poor technique resulted in unsatisfactory protection. John Simon in 1857 observed that in England and Wales there was "not only an appreciable amount of utterly incompetent vaccination but a very considerable proportion of second-rate vaccination" (6). During the epidemic of 1871 vaccination was enforced by inspectors.

This was followed by a wane in smallpox deaths (Fig. 1.2).

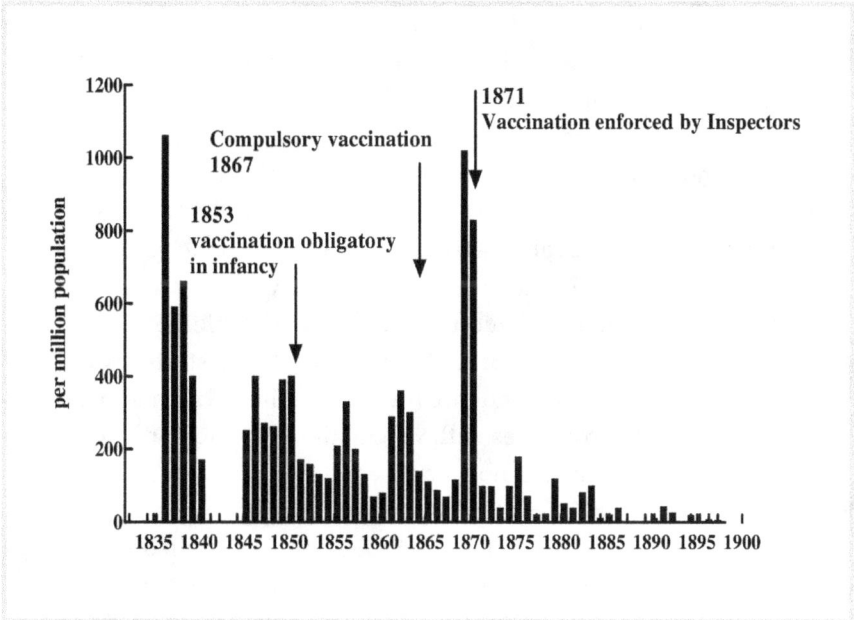

Fig. 1.2 Smallpox deaths in England, 1838-1900 (1843-1846: no reliable data available).

Austria and Belgium

Austria and Belgium had no formal vaccination policy until the last decade of the 19th century and the high mortality from smallpox reflects this.

The Attack on Vaccination

Most informed opinion would agree with the statement of Zinsser in 1931 (3) that:

> The benefits of vaccination are no longer a question of opinion, and opposition to the practice is explicable only on the basis of ignorance.

However others consider that the decline in smallpox occurred throughout Europe despite vaccination (see Ref. 4 for example). One noted opponent of animal experimentation uses carefully chosen figures of death rate from smallpox (although the actual figures are excluded from the graph) to imply that smallpox mortality was declining in England and Wales from 1840-1900 except when vaccination laws were enforced, when there was a dramatic rise (5).

Two factors have enabled those that decry the value of vaccination to muster some spurious evidence to support their claims. Firstly it was wrongly believed that inoculation with cowpox virus would provide life-long protection against smallpox (the protection lasts about ten years). Secondly was the epidemic nature of smallpox, and the fact that a devastating pandemic occurred in Europe between 1870 and 1875. The epidemic began in France and lasted about two years in each country. The occurrence of a sudden epidemic at a time when widespread vaccination was underway is eagerly seized upon as an irrefutable demonstration that vaccination was redundant. However mortality statistics for the years 1870-75 provide clear evidence for the benefits of vaccination, since mortality rates in the countries with vaccination were demonstrably less than where vaccination was not practised at that time. In England the epidemic peaked in 1871 with a death rate of 1,012 per million, in Sweden (where vaccination was started in 1801) 936 per million died in 1874. In Belgium and the Netherlands, where vaccination was not practised the rates were a striking 4,168 and 4,355 per million respectively at the height of the epidemic.

Further proof of the efficacy of vaccination (and of the necessity for revaccination) emerges from the examination of the age distribution of those dying from smallpox (data from Ref. 6). Before vaccination in England, 80% of smallpox deaths were in the younger age groups (under 10 years). As the vaccination of babies spread the ratio reversed, that is those in the older age groups formed the highest proportion of those contracting and dying of smallpox (these individuals had outgrown the immunity conferred by vaccination and of course had not acquired the long-lasting immunity secondary to a mild smallpox infection).

Were it required, additional evidence of the protection by vaccination is provided by the comparison of mortality to smallpox in adjacent countries, one of which had enforced vaccination whilst the other had not (e.g. Belgium and the Netherlands, and Austria and Bavaria).

The WHO Eradication Programme

In the first half of the twentieth century Europe and North America gradually became smallpox free due to extensive vaccination and containment measures (7). Occasional relaxation of vaccination laws always led to outbreaks which had to be suppressed by vigorous vaccination programmes. Zinsser (3) cites an outbreak in Kansas City in 1921 which led to 1,090 cases and 222 deaths. 200,000 people were vaccinated before the epidemic ceased. In 1922 in Denver there was a virulent outbreak of 805 cases with a death rate of over 30%. No order requiring vaccination was issued until November 21, 1922. The result was that there were only 81 cases in December as against 252 in November of that year.

The success of vaccination in eliminating smallpox from countries where it had been endemic raised the possibility of the global eradication of smallpox. This was proposed at the Eleventh World Health Assembly in 1958. After 8 years it was evident that technical and material assistance from the WHO would be required and this was initiated in 1967. Freeze-dried vaccine that met the WHO standards was used and a simplified vaccine technique was devised (the bifurcated needle) that made the programme easier to carry out.

Eradication programmes began in 1967, the last of the remaining 30 endemic countries to start the programme was Ethiopia in 1971 (7).

South America

In 1967 smallpox was being reported almost solely in Brazil. Over 4 years 83.3 million people were vaccinated (90% of the population). Surveillance was begun in July 1969 (which accounts for the apparent increase in incidence at that time) and in 1970 a steady decline occurred until April 1971 when the last case reported.

Africa

At the institution of the vaccination programme (1967) smallpox was endemic throughout South Saharan Africa. By 1972 smallpox incidence had decreased virtually to zero except in Sudan and Ethiopia. After 1971 vaccination and surveillance was increased in these two countries with consequent decrease in cases.

Asia (Mainland)

China had become smallpox free after extensive vaccination in the 1950s and, at the time of the eradication programme, Burma and Iran had only limited outbreaks imported from Asian countries with endemic disease – Afghanistan, India, Nepal and Pakistan.

In these endemic areas surveillance and vaccination resulted in attenuation of the disease which was somewhat slower than in other areas, due partly to the geography and partly to the persistence of variolation, which continued to be practised by itinerant shamans, particularly in Afghanistan and Pakistan.

Indonesia

The programme in Indonesia was started in July 1968 in Java and Bali and was later extended to the remaining islands. By the end of 1971 there were only a few cases in limited foci in Java and one focus in Sulawesi (see Fig. 1.3).

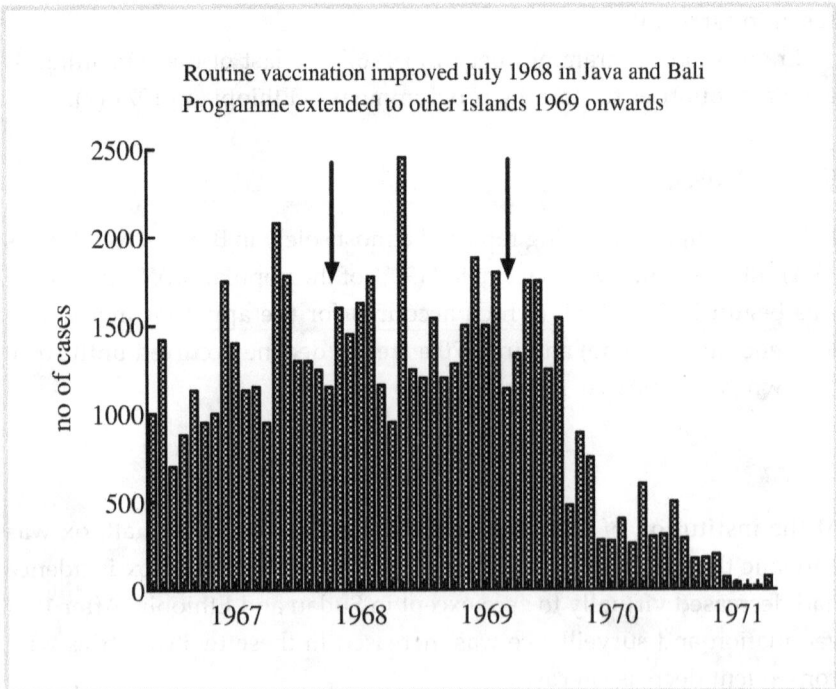

Routine vaccination improved July 1968 in Java and Bali
Programme extended to other islands 1969 onwards

Fig. 1.3 Smallpox incidence in Indonesia, 1966-1971.

Eradication

The last recorded case of smallpox was reported in Somalia in 1977 (8). In view of the long history of the disease this was an astonishing achievement which throws into sharp relief the criticisms of those who claim that vaccination was ineffective (4) and dangerous. The diminution of the disease over a hundred years in both developed and Third World countries immediately after the institution of a vaccination programme either attests to the value of the procedure or is a remarkable coincidence.

As to the dangers of vaccination, the statement by Sharpe (5) – that "vaccination was stopped in 1940 when the considerable risks were thought to outweigh the benefits" – is typical hyperbole. Serious complications of vaccination, according to the WHO (7), were so infrequent that "very large populations must be studied in order to assess the relative risks involved." In one extensive study in the USA in 1968 (7) there were 9 deaths in over 14 million vaccinations. Five of these occurred either in eczematous patients (eczema was considered a contraindication in non-endemic areas) or in patients with immunological defects.

The Scientific Origins of Immunisation

Whilst the acceptance of vaccination was spreading across Europe, Pasteur and his colleagues were carrying out experiments that were to give rise to the techniques for providing active artificial immunity to many diseases. It is of significance, and somewhat ironic, that the crucial experiments were those carried out into the cause and treatment of diseases of animals – chicken cholera and anthrax.

Chicken cholera

Chicken cholera was a lethal disease that occurred in epidemics in poultry yards. Due to the emerging prominence of the "germ theory" at that time it was thus naturally thought that the cause was a microbe. Pasteur found and described the microbe as: "tiny bodies, extremely slender and constricted in the middle, which would at first sight be taken for isolated dots."

Pasteur (Fig. 1.4) succeeded in cultivating the microbe outside the body in a neutral, sterilized broth made of ground up chicken meat. Small amounts of the broth sprinkled on the food given to chickens caused the disease, and Pasteur proceeded to demonstrate that the microbe flourished in the gut of the infected chickens, and passed on the infection through the faeces. The microbe was fatal to rabbits on inoculation but when injected into the skin of guinea pigs produced a local abscess. Such infected (but apparently generally healthy) guinea pigs however could spread the disease to both rabbits and poultry (as Pasteur remarked – how many obscurities in the history of contagions will one day be cleared up by even simpler experiments).

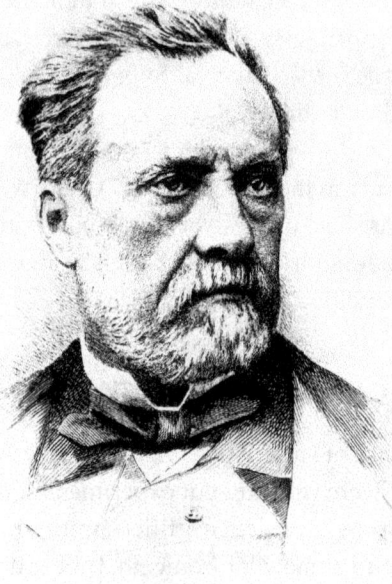

Fig. 1.4 Louis Pasteur (1822-1895), microbiologist. Wellcome Library, London, CC BY.

The crucial discovery made by Pasteur was that cultures of the chicken cholera microbes, left for some time, lost their ability to transmit the disease to hens. This was a chance observation due to cultures being left over a vacation. It was typical of the thoroughness of Pasteur that he decided to see if the "ineffective" cultures had produced any change in the condition of the chickens. On administration of a fresh culture these hens proved resistant to the disease. The same operation on hens obtained fresh from the market caused death in them all from cholera.

It was known that recurrence of a virulent disease after survival of a severe attack was rare. Resistance was conferred by the challenge. *Pasteur had found a way of producing the resistance without the risk of the disease.*

Anthrax

Although the development of a "vaccine" against chicken cholera was of enormous scientific significance the disease itself was not of great importance. Because of long experience of the disease poultry farmers kept birds in small groups and killed sick hens immediately, before the disease could spread. Anthrax on the other hand was a disease of sheep and cattle that was of enormous importance. Each year 5% of cattle and 10% of sheep died of anthrax in France. In some particular areas of France and the Argentine the mortality to farm animals was so great the land had to be left unused.

Using the culture techniques with which he had become expert Pasteur addressed the problem of the prevention of anthrax.

Small bodies, termed bacteridia, had sometimes been detected in the blood of animals suffering from anthrax, but the weight of scientific opinion considered the disease to be due to something invisible termed "virus" (as was the case for smallpox). Pasteur found that the bacteridium would grow freely in neutralised urine. By successive subculture he produced a culture diluted from the original virulent one by many million times. That this culture could still produce anthrax in guinea pigs proved that the bacteridium was the cause, since all else had been diluted out.

By a series of elegant but simple experiments Pasteur showed that the anthrax bacteridium infected sheep through the alimentary canal and also explained how the disease persisted in particular "accursed fields" (champs maudits) where cattle or sheep were bound to contract anthrax if they were allowed to graze.

Koch had shown that anthrax bacteridia could form spores in conditions of high oxygen levels and temperature. Pasteur demonstrated the presence of anthrax spores in the fine top soil of the accursed fields. The spores were brought to the surface (sometimes from the buried bodies of anthrax sheep or cattle) by earthworms. Presumably the animals ingested the anthrax spores from soil contamination of the grass or clover upon which they grazed. Extracts of the soil produced anthrax in guinea pigs even if the soil had been heated to 90°C (which kills off other soil bacteria). Pasteur also produced anthrax in guinea pigs by inoculation of the soil from the intestine of earthworms.

An Anthrax Vaccine

In order to develop an attenuated strain of bacteridia (similar to the innocuous but immunogenic culture of chicken cholera) Pasteur investigated the vitality and virulence of cultures treated in various ways. The bacteridium grew only between 16 and 44°C. When cultured at fairly high temperatures (42-43°C) a very virulent strain grew rapidly but Pasteur found that the virulence waned, so that the culture became harmless to guinea pigs after 12 days, but would kill mice. After 4 weeks even mice and baby guinea pigs survived challenge with the culture.

Pasteur was thus able to produce "vaccines" of graded strength depending upon the duration of the high temperature incubation, and he used these to protect animals against a challenge with a virulent anthrax culture. The stage was set for a field trial.

Pasteur proved the effectiveness of his vaccine with a convincing public demonstration at Pouilly-le-Fort in 1881. Under the supervision of a vet 25 sheep were inoculated with Pasteur's vaccine, 25 were not so treated. On May 31st all 50 sheep were inoculated with a virulent culture of anthrax bacteridia. The trial was a spectacular success. On June 2nd all the vaccinated sheep were in good health. Of the non-vaccinated, 22 were dead and three dying. The experiment was repeated in 10 cows with the same definitive result.

Of course criticism persisted, particularly from some veterinarians who were offended at the intrusion of a scientist in what they considered their preserve. But when the vaccine was shown also to protect animals against inoculation with blood from an animal dying from anthrax, and "not a mixture of unknown nature made up in a laboratory, and whose constitution no one knows but the makers" – all opposition disappeared.

In France, between 1882 and 1893 nearly 4 million animals received anthrax vaccine, and loss of cattle and sheep from the disease fell to low levels. The use of Pasteur's vaccine spread throughout Europe and the World. By 1914 40 million doses had been sent out from the Pasteur Institute alone.

By a simple animal experiment, of a style and to an extent that could never be reproduced in humans, Pasteur had shown indisputably that immunisation did protect against infective disease. This protection induced against an animal disease should be held as irrefutable evidence for the value of immunisation – which, of course, is repudiated by the animal rights organisations. It is also evidence that animals themselves benefit from such research. It may be alleged by opponents of animal research that protection against anthrax merely solved an economic problem for milk distributors and wool merchants. However, it undoubtedly prevented animal suffering and such a claim of vested interest cannot be levelled at the research that resulted in a vaccine that conferred protection against canine distemper.

An earlier version of this chapter was published as: Smallpox and after – an early history of the treatment and prevention of infections. *RDS News* July 1993 5-10.

References

1) De la Condamine (1759) Mémoire sur l'inoculation de la petite vérole. *Histoire et Mémoires de l'Académie Royaledes Sciences* (read at the public session of April 24, 1754).

2) Edwardes EJ (1902) *A Concise History of Small-Pox and Vaccination in Europe.* HK London: Lewis.

3) Zinsser H (1931) *Textbook of Bacteriology,* 6th edition. New York: Appleton.

4) Chaitow L (1987) *Vaccination and Immunisation: Dangers, Delusions and Alternatives.* Saffron Walden: Daniel.

5) Sharpe R (1988) *The Cruel Deception: The Use of Animals in Medical Research.* London: Thorsons.

6) Hardy A (1983) Smallpox in London: factors in the decline of the disease in the nineteenth century. *Medical History* **27** 111-38. http://dx.doi.org/10.1017/s0025727300042599

7) (1972) WHO Expert Committee on Smallpox Eradication. 2nd Report. *World Health Organization Technical Report Series* No. 493 Geneva: WHO.

8) Paton WDM (1993) *Man and Mouse.* 2nd edition, p. 77. Oxford: Oxford University Press.

Other sources

Descour L (1922) *Pasteur and his Work.* London: T Fisher Unwin.

Paget S (1914) *Pasteur and After Pasteur.* London: Black.

Duclaux E (1920) *Pasteur: The History of a Mind.* Philadelphia: Saunders.

2. Rabies

On the 17th of June, 1981 an Englishwoman travelling in India was bitten on the leg by a dog. The wound was immediately cleansed by her husband using whisky as an antiseptic. She later attended a local clinic where the wound was again washed and packed with antiseptic powder. The woman returned to England in July and the wound was redressed in her local hospital. By the middle of August she became constantly tired and complained of aches and shooting pains in the back. She was anxious and depressed, and appeared to catch her breath when trying to drink. By the 19th of August she found it impossible to drink more than a few sips. She could not bear the touch of the wind or her hair on her face and had moments of apparent terror. The following day she was confused, hallucinating, incontinent of urine and quite unable to eat or drink. For the next two days she was intermittently hallucinating and screaming with terror until she collapsed and had a cardiac arrest. Although she was resuscitated in the ambulance whilst being carried to intensive care, she died two days later, on 24th of August 1981, without recovering consciousness. The unfortunate woman had been infected by rabies virus in the saliva from the, obviously rabid, dog (Fig. 2.1). The typical symptoms and signs of rabies encephalitis that appeared two months after the initial infection had been misinterpreted as hysteria

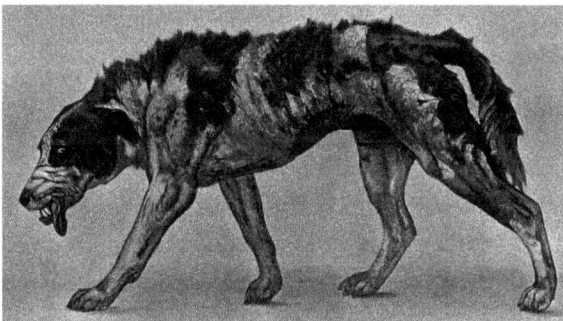

Fig. 2.1 Study of a rabid dog from an oil painting by J.T. Nettleship.
Wellcome Library, London, CC BY.

http://dx.doi.org/10.11647/OBP.0055.02

Such case reports of rabies make frightening reading. The initial phase of the disease may start some months (in some cases years) after the infected saliva has entered a puncture wound, thus the two events may not be associated. The delay is due to the slow passage of the virus along the sensory nerves to the brain and spinal cord. The initial symptoms resemble those of less serious viral diseases – weakness, headache and loss of appetite. Most patients then move into the so-called furious phase. There is an increased sensitivity to sensory stimuli and a horrifying aversion to liquids (hydrophobia), during which patients may retch and vomit so violently that the lining of the oesophagus may tear. Patients scream in alarm during periods of wild agitation, which alternate with periods of lucid calm. Eventually the patient sinks into a coma and dies. Once the central nervous system symptoms appear, death is inevitable, and the period before coma is terrifying for the patient.

Though causing the death of many wild and domesticated animals, control measures meant that rabies did not in fact kill as many people as other contagions rife until the early twentieth century. Nevertheless, because of its dreadful symptoms, it has been called "the most severe of all the communicable diseases." (1)

Rabies is still endemic in most parts of the world. Its incidence is under-reported partly for political reasons, and partly because it may be unsuspected as a cause of death. In India, Pakistan and Bangladesh there may have been as many as 50,000 deaths per year in the 1970s (2). Sri Lanka, The Philippines and Thailand each lose approximately 1,000 citizens per year due to rabies and the incidence of the disease is also high in China, Iran and Colombia.

Rabies in Britain

In Britain rabies was certainly known in 1000 AD and probably much earlier. In the mid-eighteenth century the situation was so bad that a two shilling reward (then a considerable sum) was offered for the destruction of each stray dog. In the early nineteenth century, packs of hounds had to be destroyed (including the Quorn, a well-known hunt in England) and 36 persons were alleged to die annually from rabies, although this was probably an underestimate.

Outbreaks of rabies continued throughout the nineteenth century in various centres in Britain, and thousands of rabid animals, mainly dogs, were destroyed (Fig. 2.2). By 1864 rabies was widespread in animals in and around London. The Metropolitan Streets Act was passed in 1867, enabling police to seize all vagrant dogs, and rabies then declined (2).

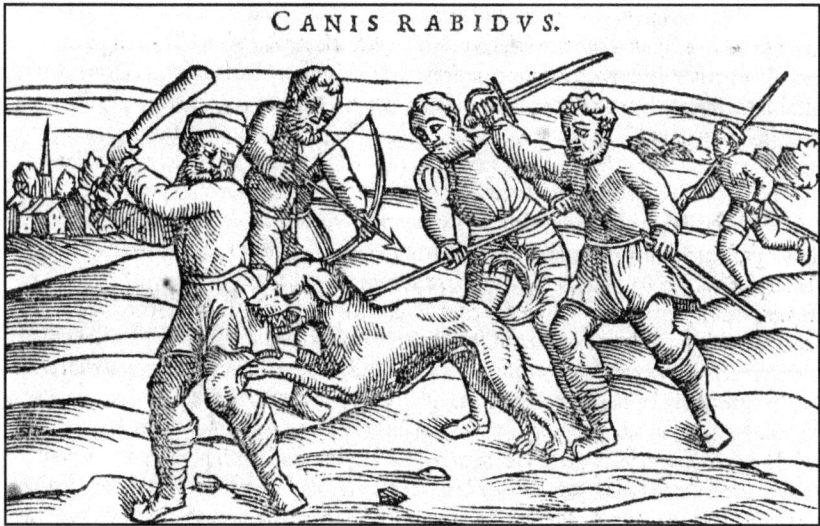

Fig. 2.2 Slaying of a rabid dog. Wellcome Library, London, CC BY.

Due to the imposition of strict quarantine laws, rabies was eradicated from Britain in 1903 (There was however an outbreak that originated in Plymouth in 1918 from a dog illegally brought back from the continent. About 300 dogs became infected and 358 persons had to be given anti-rabies treatment (3)).

Rabies in Europe

In the nineteenth century rabies was widespread in Continental Europe, with extensive outbreaks occurring in various species. In an outbreak in 1803, many people, dogs and pigs were bitten by rabid foxes in France, and the foothills of the Jura Alps were littered with the bodies of rabid animals. Between 1800 and 1841, 800 dogs had died of rabies in the veterinary hospital at Lyon alone. By the middle of the century, 60% of the dogs taken to this hospital were rabid (2).

Bites from rabid wolves were commonplace. In 1851 a single rabid wolf bit 46 persons and 82 head of cattle in one day in the vicinity of Hue-Au-Gal. Many people died and all the cattle had to be destroyed (2). By 1869 rabies had become common even in large towns. In that year a rabid cat passed on the disease to a woman in Paris.

Pasteur and his Research on Rabies

Against this background of rabies endemic in the woods, mountains and by then even the large cities of France, Pasteur launched his researches into the nature and treatment of the disease. Pasteur had up to 1880 worked on the prevention of animal diseases but had always intended to seek "the causes of putrid and contagious diseases that affect man."(4)

Rabies, an animal disease transmissible to humans, was thus an eminently suitable field of research. Pasteur also had had an early experience of the horror of rabies. As an eight-year-old boy he had witnessed victims of the bite of a rabid wolf arriving at the blacksmith's forge in his home town of Arbois in eastern France, to have their wounds cauterised (5). A procedure of doubtful value but the sole preventive treatment for rabies at that time.

Pasteur was convinced that rabies did not occur spontaneously in dogs, but that each case derived from another. Obvious today, this view was not commonly held in the 1880s. The saliva of rabid animals was an obvious source of the infective organism and Pasteur attempted to infect rabbits by inoculation of saliva from patients dying of rabies. He also, with some bravery, collected saliva from rabid dogs for the same purpose. The deliberately infected animals died. From his researches, Pasteur did not believe that any of the visible micro-organisms in saliva were the cause of rabies, nor was he convinced that the rabbits always died of rabies (rabbits with rabies sink into a "painless kind of paralysis" rather than the "rage" seen in dogs (4)). Further, the latent period before the disease became evident varied tremendously, making the experiments long and unpredictable.

It is tempting to believe that Pasteur sensed intuitively that the sometimes very long incubation period of rabies was because the infective organism took a long time to reach the central nervous system via the peripheral nerves. At all events, Pasteur decided that using the brain and spinal cord of infected animals was the best way of transmitting the disease for his particular experimental purposes.

Placement of portions of the brain of a dog dead from rabies under the skin of rabbits reliably produced the disease, but there was still a prolonged latent period. The crucial experiment was to place the infected tissue onto the surface of the brain of rabbits. This was achieved by removal of a small disc of bone from the skull of a rabbit under chloroform anaesthesia and placing the infected brain tissue just under the membrane surrounding the brain (the dura). This technique always resulted in the production of rabies within 20 days. Pasteur shortened the incubation period to 6-7 days by increasing the virulence of the virus, as he had previously done with anthrax, by repetitive passage through rabbits. Thus, Pasteur had prepared a very active virus with an absolutely predictable ability to cause the disease within a short time (he termed this his *virus fixe*). The way was now open to explore methods to attenuate the virus, as Pasteur had done with the microorganisms responsible for chicken cholera and anthrax.

Pasteur's Vaccine

Pasteur removed the spinal cord of a rabbit killed by the *virus fixe* and stored it in an aseptic flask in dried, filtered air in the dark at constant temperature. Under these conditions, portions of the cord gradually lost their ability to infect until, after 12 days, they appeared innocuous. By inoculating many rabbits at different times, Pasteur was able to collect a series of cords ranging in potency from the ineffectual to the highly virulent. Dogs were inoculated with portions of the cords suspended in a small volume of broth, starting with a non-virulent sample and gradually, over 12 days or so, using samples of increasing virulence until the dogs were ultimately shown to be resistant to challenge with the *virus fixe*. Pasteur demonstrated that 50 dogs so treated were unaffected by bites from rabid dogs and were even resistant to administration of the *virus fixe* to the surface of the brain. Early this century, modifications of the Pasteur vaccine were used to vaccinate dogs. A consequent fall in the incidence of canine rabies was reported from Morocco, Hungary, Finland, Algeria, Yugoslavia and various parts of the USA (6).

The most intense canine vaccination programme was started in Japan in 1918. From 1921, a phenol-inactivated virus prepared by Fermi was used as a vaccine. By 1934 1.5 million dogs had been vaccinated. The annual number of rabies cases in dogs dropped from 1,041 in 1918 to 60 in 1930 (6). In the 1950s, vaccination was made compulsory and all stray and feral dogs were seized and destroyed. As a result, the last case of canine rabies in Japan occurred in 1956, though the disease had existed there since the 10th century (2).

Treatment of Human Rabies

The *virus fixe* vaccine of Pasteur was potentially too toxic for routine prophylaxis in humans. At the outset of his researches into rabies Pasteur had suggested that, because of the long incubation period, protection by vaccination might be possible *after* the bite of a rabid animal. He obtained evidence for this by allowing pairs of dogs to be bitten by a rabid animal; one was then vaccinated the other untreated. In each case the untreated dog died, the vaccinated animal lived.

Not everyone accepts that the experimental studies proved that post-exposure vaccination was effective in preventing rabies. Webster (7) considers that all the early studies (including those of Pasteur) were faulted by poor controls. The studies of Fermi, who used a simpler, phenol inactivated virus as a vaccine, are however generally accepted as demonstrating a post-exposure prophylaxis.

Notwithstanding the subsequent debate over the experimental studies, it is difficult not to accept that post-exposure prophylaxis developed by Pasteur was beneficial in humans. The first patient publicly recorded as being treated by Pasteur probably provides the best known case history in medicine. Joseph Meister, a nine-year-old from Alsace, was brought to Pasteur on July 6th 1885. He had been attacked on July 4th by a dog, thrown to the ground and bitten fourteen times. When found, his wounds were covered with the animal's saliva. The dog subsequently attacked his owner and was shot; the body had shown evidence of rabies (2).

Pasteur and his colleagues decided that they must treat the boy, since the extent and nature of the wounds meant he was highly likely to develop rabies. 60 hours after the attack, Joseph Meister was injected with an infected cord that had been desiccated for 15 days. He received 13 injections over the next 10 days, the final injection being a virulent sample. The boy survived and was subsequently employed at the Pasteur Institute.

Three months later a second patient was successfully treated and the news of these two successes, which spread with remarkable rapidity, resulted in a steady flow of potential rabies cases to Paris. In 1886 Pasteur reported the results of treating 350 cases of rabies. Only one had died, a child whose treatment was delayed 5 weeks after being bitten. The most conservative contemporary statistics as to the likelihood of rabies developing after dog bites in Paris range from 16 to 40 per hundred persons bitten (8), although some authorities claim the figure was 50% (2).

By the end of 1886, 2,000 people had been treated, including 38 Russians bitten by rabid wolves (three of these died, bites from rabid wolves having a particularly high mortality). Pasteur noted however, that the treatment was not always successful, particularly when the face was bitten. Nonetheless, the value of Pasteur's crude vaccine can be assessed by examination of the detailed reports that appeared each year from the Pasteur Institute. In 1898 Pottevin reported a total of 20,166 patients treated at the Pasteur Institute with only 96 deaths – a mortality of 0.48% (2).

Criticisms by the Antivivisectionists

Pasteur's researches were acclaimed, and not only within France. In 1886 the British government appointed a Committee to examine Pasteur's method; it reported favourably and in 1889 a donation of 40,000 francs was made by the government to the Pasteur Institute (4). Anti-rabic institutes, using the Pasteur technique, were opened in many parts of the world.

There is no doubt that contemporary opinion regarded the experimental work on rabies as prodigious. It is sad that a century later, those that seek to belittle the contribution of animal experimentation to medical progress find it necessary to disparage a researcher of the stature of Pasteur. Thus one critic states that Pasteur's vaccine "turned out to be a failure." (9) His attempted justification is the uncertainty that rabies will inevitably follow a bite from a rabid animal, implying that in the early clinical studies those that were inoculated after a bite would not have developed rabies anyway.

Obviously a controlled trial, whereby vaccine treatment is deliberately withheld from some patients, would be unethical. Thus the only way to assess the effectiveness of the vaccine is to examine data of the incidence of rabies following bites before development of the vaccine, or data from studies where patients refused the vaccine. Fleming, in 1872 (10) described the clinical course of 198 patients bitten by rabid dogs. Of 132 who had the wound cauterised, 41 died (31%), of the remaining 66 that were not cauterised, 55 died (84%). The mortality in treated patients after the development of the vaccine was between 0.2 and 1.3%.

The most emphatic data was that recorded by the Pasteur Institute of Southern India, Madras (11). Of 28,898 cases treated over 16 years, 0.7% were treatment failures. Of 423 persons bitten by rabid dogs in Madras and who received no treatment, 148 died of hydrophobia – a 35% mortality.

There is little doubt that the vaccine was effective, but by modern day standards it was certainly not safe. Even the later phenol or glycerin-treated vaccines, because of their high nerve-protein content, caused severe neurological complications for 1 in 2,000 patients (2).

Due to the remarkable progress in the prevention and treatment of disease over the last 100 years, patients today enjoy a high expectation of safe treatment. Thus the dangers of the early anti-rabies vaccines now seem grievous. This is another reason that their value, and hence the significance of the experiments that produced them, is peremptorily dismissed in animal rights propaganda.

It should require (for the unbiased reader) only a superficial examination of contemporary records to understand the import of Pasteur's research. A horrific and inevitably fatal disease had but one treatment – vaccination. Despite its risks, at the time such treatment was not only acceptable but eagerly sought.

Local Wound Treatment

Even 2,000 years ago it was realised that bite wounds from rabid animals were probably the portal of entry of the factor responsible for rabies. Irrigation of the wounds with various noxious substances and cauterization were common until the availability of standard viral preparations enabled experimental studies to be undertaken to establish optimum wound treatment. These studies are well reviewed by Cabasso (2). Typically, guinea pigs were infected with the virus through a wound in the neck or hind limb, or mice had the virus implanted in the hind-limb or foot pad. The effectiveness of various techniques in preventing the development of the disease was then assessed.

Fortunately, the earliest studies resulted in the rejection of cauterization and fuming nitric acid to irrigate the wound (these techniques were common even in the early 20th century). Washing with 20% soap solution was found as effective as these traumatic and painful measures. Of the many other chemicals used in the experimental studies, quaternary ammonium compounds were found to be valuable, with benzalkonium chloride being particularly effective. Of some practical significance, ethyl alcohol was surprisingly efficacious even in concentrations as low as 20%.

The present recommended wound treatment in humans stems from these animal studies. Dead tissue should be removed and the wound flushed with soapy water or a 1-2% solution of benzalkonium chloride. If the wound is deep the viricidal benzalkonium chloride must be used, if it is not available then 40-70% ethyl alcohol is the best alternative. Passive immunisation with anti-rabies antibodies is also used.

Passive Immunisation

Since vaccination results in the production of antibodies in the treated person, it was not surprising that immune serum, i.e. serum from vaccinated animals, was tested to see whether it could protect infected animals.

Habel in 1945 (described in Ref. 2) obtained a serum from rabbits hyper-immunised with mouse brain fixed virus. Given to guinea pigs previously infected with rabies the antiserum had a significant, dose-dependent protective effect, the benefit being greatest if the antiserum was given soon after infection. Similar protection was seen in mice challenged with mouse-adapted virus where the development of rabies was prevented if the serum was given within three hours.

These experimental studies were confirmed and extended by Koprowski (12) who raised anti-rabies antibodies in rabbits and sheep to protect infected hamsters. Koprowski also made the highly significant observation that small doses of anti-rabies globulin and vaccine given together completely protected guinea pigs against rabies, whereas given alone they were ineffective. This apparent synergistic effect of the vaccine and anti-rabies serum was followed up by the World Health Organisation's Expert Committee on Rabies, which instituted a field trial with vaccine and anti-rabies antibodies raised in horses (anti-rabies equine serum). The test was carried out in Iran where there was a high fatality rate amongst humans bitten by wolves. Careful, controlled studies such as those of Koprowski cannot ethically be carried out in humans, nonetheless the few cases initially treated were encouraging. In 1954 a chance of obtaining definitive evidence arose when a rabid wolf entered a village and bit 29 persons. The wounds were all severe. A six-year-old boy was bitten in the head, his skull was partially crushed and penetrated deeply by the wolf's teeth; he presented with meningeal lesions and convulsions.

Of the 17 patients given antiserum plus vaccine, one died (6%). Of those with severe head wounds given vaccine only, 75% died. The boy with the crushed skull was given six injections of the equine antiserum and, remarkably, was one of the survivors (2). Serological tests on all the victims confirmed emphatically that concurrent use of antiserum greatly increased the beneficial effects of the vaccine. Combined use of anti-rabies antibodies with the modern vaccines is now routine for post-exposure prophylaxis against rabies, as is administration of the antibody preparations to the potentially infected wound.

Modern Vaccines and Immunotherapy

As indicated previously, useful as the nervous tissue vaccine was, it was not without risk, particularly because of its nerve-protein content. Improvement in safety was achieved firstly by the culture of the virus in embryonated hen or duck eggs (1940-56) and then by culture on hamster kidney cells (1960). Though such vaccines were free of protein of nervous origin they still contained potentially harmful factors (2). The development of the human diploid cell (HDC) line provided an improved method of culturing the virus and preparing the safest vaccine (HDCV), which was first used in Iran in 1972.

Similarly, the equine antiserum, though dramatically effective when used in conjunction with the vaccine, could cause anaphylactic shock in a few patients (although the possibility of this occurring could be tested by conjunctival or intradermal administration of a small amount of serum). Hence today rabies immune globulin of human origin (RIGH) is available. This is obtained from immunised donors by repeated bleedings, using plasmaphaeresis, whereby whole blood is removed, the cells separated from the plasma (retained for patient use), resuspended in saline and reinfused into the donor (2).

We have thus perfected the treatment of rabies. Today post-infection prophylaxis is effective and safe, using vaccines grown on human cells and antisera obtained from human plasma. Objectors to animal experiments use this fact to dismiss the contribution of the early animal experiments to the treatment of rabies. This is at best naive. Modern experimenters have been able to refine treatments using modern techniques and human tissue because they could harvest the yield of the experiments of giants such as Pasteur and his colleagues.

Rabies Eradication?

A significant step towards the possible eradication of rabies is the development of a novel vaccine using *vaccinia virus* (which was responsible for smallpox eradication). The vaccine is produced by inserting the gene coding for the protein conferring immunity to rabies into the genome of *vaccinia virus* (VV). The modified VV is used to infect cultured cells which correctly express the rabies antigen. This antigen has potently induced rabies virus-neutralising antibodies in rabbits and mice and protected the animals against challenge with a lethal strain of rabies virus (13).

This vaccine is active orally and has been used in bait to immunise raccoons in the USA and foxes in Europe. Innocuous to mammals, the vaccine is undergoing field trials in Belgium and France. Widespread immunisation of feral and domesticated animals would be the first step towards the ultimate eradication of rabies.

An earlier version of this chapter was published as: Rabies – a century of research brings eradication closer. *RDS News* October 1993 8-12.

References

1) Kaplan C, Turner G & Warrell D (1986) *Rabies: The Facts*. Oxford: Oxford University Press.

2) Baer G M (ed) (1991) *The Natural History of Rabies*. 2nd edition. Boca Raton: CRC Press.

3) Anon. The menace of rabies. *The Lancet* (1944) **244** 6324 628-29.

4) Paget S (1914) *Pasteur and after Pasteur*. London: Black.

5) Geison G (1995) *The Private Science of Louis Pasteur*. Princeton: Princeton University Press p. 17.

6) Rogers L (1937) *The Truth About Vivisection*. London: Churchill.

7) Webster L (1939) The immunizing potency of antirabies vaccines. A critical review. *Am J Hygiene* **30** 113-34.

8) Weatherall M (1990) *In Search of a Cure: A History of Pharmaceutical Discovery*. Oxford: Oxford University Press.

9) Sharpe R (1988) *The Cruel Deception: The Use of Animals in Medical Research*. London: Thorsons.

10) Fleming G (1872) *Rabies and Hydrophobia*. London: Chapman & Hall.

11) Statistics of antirabies inoculations in India. *BMJ* (1923) Aug 18 p. 298. http://www.bmj.com/content/2/3268/298.1

12) Koprowski H, Van der Sheer J & Black J (1950) Use of hyperimmune antirabies serum concentrates in experimental rabies. *Am J Med* 8 412. http://dx.doi.org/10.1016/0002-9343(50)90224-5

13) Cryz S J (ed) (1991) *Vaccines and Immunotherapy*. New York: Pergamon.

3. Lockjaw: Prevalent but Preventable

Tetanus is one of the most dreadful diseases which has been produced in nature to torment mankind. No one who has seen a case can ever forget it. The poor victim, thrown every few minutes into the most violent spasms, bent backwards to such an extent that only his head and heels touch the bed, his teeth tightly clenched, unable to eat or drink, his face expressing the fiendish torture he is undergoing, at last is mercifully released by death.

Sir David Bruce (1920) (1)

Although tetanus was described at the time of Hippocrates, for over 2000 years there was no advance in our understanding of the disease. At the end of the nineteenth century the prevalent, rather naive view was that it was caused by "inflammation travelling up an injured nerve to the central nervous system." (2)

The infective nature of tetanus was demonstrated by Carle and Rattone, who in 1884 took pus from a lesion of a patient with tetanus and injected it into rabbits, where it produced signs typical of the disease (3).

The Causative Organism

Tetanus frequently followed wounds where the skin had been deeply punctured, particularly if the lesions were contaminated with soil or other foreign matter such as splinters etc. Nicolaier, in 1884, established that the infective organism was present in the soil. He produced the disease in mice, rabbits and guinea pigs by inoculation of various samples of soil under the skin (4). Soil from richly manured areas, such as grazing land and the ground around stables, was particularly potent.

http://dx.doi.org/10.11647/OBP.0055.03

The identification of the bacterium responsible for tetanus was delayed because of the enormous variety of organisms present in manure-contaminated soil. Kitasato in 1889, provided definitive evidence of the identity of the causative bacterium by the use of heat (80^0 for one hour) to destroy non spore-bearing organisms, followed by culture in the absence of oxygen. The pure culture of "drumstick-like" anaerobic bacteria (subsequently known as *Clostridium tetani*) produced the typical symptoms of tetanus on inoculation into animals (5).

Tetanus Toxin

As with diphtheria, the tetanus bacillus is not invasive. It stays in the area of damage, grows and exudes a toxin which produces the symptoms of the disease. Bacteria-free filtrates of broth cultures, prepared according to the method of Kitasato, were shown to be potently toxic to animals, a few hundredths of a microlitre proving fatal to mice of 10g body weight (6).

The absorption of the toxin accounts for all the pathology of tetanus. In animals, after a latent period of 1 to 3 days, spasm occurs in the muscles at the site of the inoculation. However, should the toxin be administered intravenously, generalised muscle spasm occurs (7). This suggested that the toxin exerts its action in the central nervous system having reached there by transport along the motor nerves. This was proved by Bruschettini (8) who showed that toxin injected into muscle in rabbit could be recovered from motor nerves supplying that area. Similar animal experiments demonstrated that toxin injected into the sciatic nerve could, after a period, be recovered from the spinal cord of the animal. The fact that "local tetanus" in animals could be prevented by sclerosis or actual section of the nerve, confirmed that passage along motor nerves lying near to the focus of the tetanus infection was the means by which the toxin entered the central nervous system, where it caused its toxic actions. These experiments had profound implications for the use, and the route of administration, of the antitoxin which was developed later.

Tetanus Antitoxin

In view of the scientific climate in the late 19th century it was predictable that researchers should try to ascertain if animals could be stimulated to produce a substance that could neutralise tetanus toxin, and thus combat tetanus infection. It was perhaps also predictable that the production of a tetanus antitoxin in animals (after serial injections of gradually increasing amounts of tetanus bacillus filtrates) was demonstrated by von Behring and Kitasato, who also produced the diphtheria antitoxin (9). The antitoxin was able to protect animals against large doses of tetanus toxin or large numbers of tetanus bacilli.

Toxin was obtained by filtration of suitable cultures. The potency of the toxin was standardised by making serial dilutions and determining the minimal lethal dose (MLD) after subcutaneous injection into white mice of 20g body weight. Multiples of this MLD, perhaps rendered less noxious by treatment with terchloride of iodine, were administered to a horse in increasing doses at intervals of 8 days or more. Eventually the horse had generated sufficient antibody to withstand challenge with very high doses of tetanus toxin. The antitoxic serum was obtained by bleeding from the jugular vein and was preserved with small concentrations of phenol or tricresol. The preparation was standardised by measurement of the volume needed to protect animals (mice or guinea pigs) against lethal doses of toxin, and diluting the antitoxin solution accordingly (7).

Prophylaxis with Antitoxin

It soon became clear from experimental studies that tetanus antitoxin could only neutralise toxin that had not yet entered the motor nerves. Roux and Borrel in 1898 (10) demonstrated that rabbits with sufficient antibody in their plasma to protect them from huge doses of tetanus toxin given intravenously, readily succumbed to minute doses of toxin given by intracerebral injection. Nevertheless much animal data attested to the prophylactic value of tetanus antitoxin. The horse is particularly susceptible to tetanus infection, and tetanus following surgery or injection in this animal was commonplace. There were many reports at the turn of the century as to the prophylactic value of tetanus antiserum in the horse. A study on several hundred horses used for the production of various antisera in a large laboratory in the USA showed a 10% death-rate from tetanus despite rigid aseptic technique and disinfection. After routine prophylactic use of antitoxin before any surgical procedure, death-rate was reduced to 1% (2)

Antitoxin Prophylaxis in Humans

Although hundreds of thousands still die from tetanus infection each year, it was during war that deaths from tetanus reached epidemic proportions. Missiles such as musket balls, bullets or shrapnel, blasted through soil-contaminated clothing produce the deeply penetrating wounds in which *clostridium tetani* bacteria flourish. Thus military medicine provides the first clinical evidence for the efficacy of tetanus antitoxin.

According to Larrey, in Napoleon's campaign the tetanus case mortality was 82% (cited in 1). During the American civil war case mortality was 89.3% (11, p. 203), 82% during the Franco-Prussian war of 1871 (on the German side) (1) and 90% on the British side in the Crimean war (1). The 1914-18 war was the first real testing ground for the then freely available tetanus antiserum (Fig. 3.1).

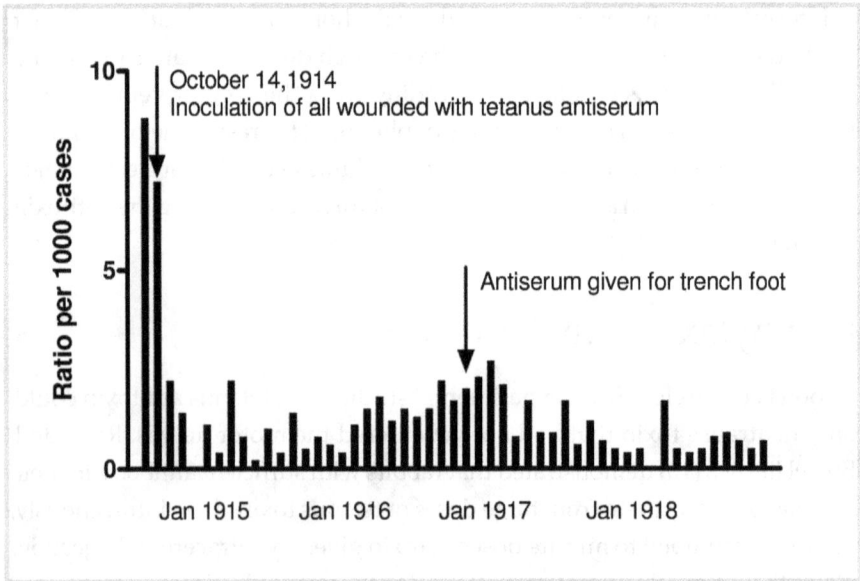

Fig. 3.1 Incidence of tetanus per 1,000 wounded in the British Army, 1914-1918.

Evidence from animal studies that the antitoxin would be effective as prophylaxis against tetanus was clear. Faced with evidence of a tetanus case mortality averaging 85%, one might have expected the British Army Medical Service in 1914 to have recommended routine administration of the antiserum to all wounded personnel. This was not the case however. For almost the first two months of the war no antiserum was used, with the result that incidence of tetanus was high. The reason for this lapse of clinical judgement was that the most recent experience of the traumas of active service was that of the Boer War. Tetanus during that campaign was rare since the veldt was clean, unlike the highly cultivated soil of Northern Europe. Although this error undoubtedly caused needless deaths during the first few weeks of the war, it also provided evidence of the clinical benefit of the antitoxin through the dramatic fall in incidence of tetanus after the belated adoption of routine anti-tetanus prophylaxis (1).

Evidence for the value of tetanus antitoxin in preventing the development of tetanus after serious wounds is undoubted, although never in fact subjected to definitive test. Without question, in medical units where *all* wounded were given antitoxin at the moment of entry to the field hospital, the incidence of tetanus was at most one third of that where the antitoxin was given only where the case was considered "suspicious"(12). Bazy describes a clinical situation involving 200 soldiers with similar wounds, where "on account of certain circumstances" (unspecified by the author) only 100 received antitoxin. Of these, only one developed tetanus, and that very soon after the injection, suggesting that the disease had already taken hold. Of the 100 left unprotected, 18 developed tetanus. Thus the "certain circumstances" that obtained in Bazy's study, whilst unfortunate for 18 subjects, provided something akin to a partially controlled clinical trial to demonstrate the efficacy of tetanus antitoxin (12).

Therapy with Antitoxin

The value of antitoxin to treat tetanus once the central nervous effects of the disease are manifest is less easy to establish. The heterogeneity amongst patients with tetanus and the ethical problem of withholding a potentially life-saving treatment mean that a properly controlled trial is hard to conduct. One such, assessed by sequential analysis, did show a significant benefit from administration of 200,000 units of antitoxin (13). The small number of patients in this trial (38 pairs) has meant that the results are not accepted everywhere.

In view of the knowledge of the nature of the progress of infection by tetanus (derived solely from animal experiments) one might have supposed that injection of antitoxin direct into the nervous system would be attempted, since this is where the toxin is exerting its pathological effects. Indeed, in a particularly rigorous experiment, Sherrington (14) showed that intrathecal injection of antiserum to rhesus monkeys could reduce mortality to a substantial dose of toxin from 100% to 48%, even if the injection of the antidote was delayed until overt signs of tetanus were apparent.

It appears, however, that physicians were loath to administer a foreign protein (i.e. equine antitoxin) into the human central nervous system. Some trials carried out in India (15) demonstrated that the equine antitoxin given intrathecally was beneficial if administered less than 24 hours after start of symptoms, and a report from Irwin Hospital showed that intrathecal injection of human tetanus immune globulin reduced mortality from "mild" tetanus from 21% to 2% (15).

It is clear that tetanus antitoxin is prophylactic if administered in repeated doses to patients at risk of infection. However, once the disease has taken hold, antitoxin will be of use only to neutralize toxin that has not yet entered the nervous system, or if given intrathecally, to negate the effect of toxin that is in the nervous system but not yet fixed to the tissues. Complete control of the disease could only be achieved by effective immunisation programmes.

Immunisation against Tetanus

Effective immunisation against tetanus became possible when Descombey (16) demonstrated that tetanus toxin was rendered innocuous after prolonged incubation with formaldehyde (thus forming "toxoid"). Bergey and Etris (17) showed that three doses of toxoid, given over a period, could protect guinea pigs against injection of several thousand times a lethal dose of tetanus toxin. Since the 1930s toxoid, or toxoid precipitated with alum or other agents, has been widely used in humans.

Preparation of Toxoid

Tetanus vaccine is prepared as prescribed by the World Health Organisation (18). Tetanus toxin is obtained from a liquid medium in which a high-yielding strain of *clostridium tetani* has been cultured. The toxin is converted to the non-toxic "toxoid" by treatment with a dilute solution of formaldehyde for days or weeks. During this time the product is continually tested for toxicity in animals. The complete conversion of toxin to toxoid is established by injection of suitably diluted samples into 5 guinea pigs. The sample of toxoid passes this formal "specific toxicity test" if no guinea pig shows sign of paralysis or any other sign of tetanus within 21 days. Potency tests (protection of guinea pigs against challenge with a subcutaneous injection) and a test for innocuity (intraperitoneal injection to mice and guinea pigs) are also stipulated by the WHO monograph and national pharmacopoeias.

The Success of Tetanus Immunisation

Routine vaccination against tetanus has been the norm in developed countries for three or four decades. Effectiveness of the procedure is generally assessed by the presence of high antibody titres in the blood. Due to the consequent rarity of the condition in the developed world, as with antitoxin, one has to look to war to provide evidence of the efficacy of vaccination.

Unfortunately, during war reliable data is not always accurately recorded. Nevertheless a good account of the incidence of tetanus in the US Army is reported by Long and Sartwell (19). All US troops were immunised with tetanus toxoid from 1941. During World War I, when troops were non-immunised, out of 523,158 wounded 70 developed tetanus. During World War II 2,734,819 soldiers were wounded, yet only 12 cases of tetanus occurred, and six of these occurred in subjects who were not in fact immunised, for a variety of administrative reasons. In the Pacific theatre incidence of tetanus was high amongst non-immunised troops and civilians. In a group of 550 wounded Japanese prisoners of war in the Marshall Islands, 26 developed tetanus, and tetanus caused approximately 400 deaths of civilians injured in the war zones of Manilla and Saipan. Other comparative data attest to the protective value of vaccination against tetanus (20, 21)

Neonatal Tetanus

Current estimates of mortality from tetanus are 800,000 deaths per year from neonatal tetanus, and 120,000 to 300,000 deaths from non-neonatal tetanus (22). The cause of neonatal tetanus is generally due to infection of the umbilical scar caused by poor obstetric technique. Tetanus accounts for approximately 50% of neonatal deaths and 25% of infant deaths (22). As noted by Habig and Tankersley, "this high incidence is additionally tragic because the disease is largely preventable by appropriate immunisation." (23)

Conclusive proof of the value of tetanus toxoid in the prevention of tetanus is provided by a double-blind controlled field trial for the prevention of tetanus neonatorum in Colombia (South America), where in 1966 the estimated death rate from the condition was 11.6 per 100 births. Over 2.5 thousand women were initially involved in the trial. The control group received injection of a polyvalent influenza-virus vaccine, the test group aluminium-phosphate-adsorbed tetanus toxoid. In children born to women in the control group, incidence of neonatal tetanus was 7.8 per 100 births

(27/347). None of the 341 children born to mothers previously given 2 or 3 doses of tetanus toxoid developed the disease. Non-tetanus mortality in the two groups was similar (5.5 and 4.1% respectively) (24, Table 1).

THE USE OF TETANUS TOXOID FOR THE PREVENTION OF NEONATAL TETANUS.
Report of a double-blind controlled field trial covering 1618 women in a rural area of Colombia.
From Newell, Duenas Lehmann, Leblanc & Garces Osorio (1966) *Bulletin of the WHO* 35 863-71.

	Control	Vaccinated
Total births	347	341
Tetanus mortality (%)	27 (7.8)	0 (0)
Non-tetanus mortality (%)	19 (5.5)	14 (4.1)

Management of Tetanus

Knowledge obtained through animal experimentation has not only contributed to development of tetanus antitoxin and toxoid, but also to other modes of treatment. Antibiotics (penicillin and metronidazole) may be given to prevent the growth of *clostridium tetani* and so prevent further accumulation of toxin. Should the disease have taken hold and convulsions started, neuromuscular blocking drugs must be used to prevent spasm, and breathing maintained by positive pressure ventilation (25). The development of both antibiotics and neuromuscular blocking drugs depended totally on animal experimentation.

The Action of Tetanus Toxin

Many potent toxins of plant and animal origin have proved to be valuable tools to elucidate cell and organ function. Botulinus toxin and black widow spider venom are two notable examples. Tetanus toxin is no exception. It has been shown to prevent the release of chemical transmitters from nerves by a highly selective action on a protein present in the outer membrane of the vesicle that encloses the stores of transmitter in nerve endings. Presumably the toxin has a particular affinity for those nerves in the spinal cord that release inhibitory transmitters. Disruption of activity of these nerves would cause overactivity of motor nerves and generalised spasm. Recent research in rat tissue (26) shows that tetanus toxin is a zinc endopeptidase enzyme that selectively destroys the membrane protein, synaptobrevin. Use of the toxin will help to unravel the various functions of the different constituents of the vesicular membrane. With such tools we shall eventually elucidate the esoteric, intracellular processes controlling the storage and release of chemical messengers from nerve cells. We may also, incidentally, expose new methods of treatments for tetanus, for example the use of zinc endopeptidase inhibitors such as the antihypertensive drug, captopril.

Tetanus toxin was isolated 30 years before chemical transmission of nerve action was even raised as a possibility. The fact that some 60 years on, we are anticipating the use of this toxin in the elucidation of intricate molecular processes governing release of neurotransmitters from individual nerve cells is an example of the remarkable exponential nature of the progress of research.

Tetanus Today

Tetanus still occurs, even in developed countries. Typically it strikes females over 50 years of age, frequently infected after a minor cut or abrasion sustained while gardening. This susceptibility is due to the fact that routine tetanus immunisation of infants began only in the 1950s. Thus, those too old to have benefited from this, and who did not receive the vaccine as a member of the armed forces, would be vulnerable. Three recent cases have been reported in patients over 60 (27). This argues for vaccination for those unprotected and who are at risk by virtue of their job or hobby.

Tetanus vaccination appears to have been ignored by the animal rights lobby. No attack upon its usefulness can be found after a brief examination of recent antivivisection literature. This is probably due to its undoubted efficacy, its remarkable safety (side effects are virtually non-existent) and to its widespread use to protect animals against the disease. *The Index of Veterinary Specialities* lists 20 vaccine preparations containing tetanus toxoid, alone or in combination with vaccines against other animal diseases (28).

An earlier version of this chapter was published as: Lockjaw: prevalent but preventable. *RDS News* April 1994 6-9.

References

1) Bruce D (1920) *The Prevention of Tetanus during the Great War by the Use of Antitetanic Serum*. London: Pulman & Sons.

2) Paget S (1906) *Experiments on Animals*. 3rd ed London: James Nesbit & Co.

3) Carle and Rattone (1884) *Giornale dell'Accademia di Medicina di Torino*. 3rd series **32** 174.

4) Nicolaier A (1884) Ueber infectiösen Tetanus. *Deutsch Med Woch* **10** 842-44. http://dx.doi.org/10.1055/s-0028-1143432

5) Kitasato S (1889) Ueber den Tetanusbacillus. *Zeit fur Hyg* **7** 225-34. http://dx.doi.org/10.1007/BF02188336

6) Brieger and Cohn, cited in Zinsser H (1931) *Textbook of Bacteriology*. 6th edition New York: Appleton.

7) Zinsser (as above).

8) Bruschettini A (1890) Diffusione negli organi del veleno tetano. *Riforma Medica* **6** 1346.

9) Von Behring E & Kitasato S (1890) The mechanism of diphtheria and tetanus immunity in animals. *Deutsch Med Woch* **16** 1113.

10) Roux E & Borrel A (1898) Tétanos cérébral et immunité contre le tétanos. *Annales de l'Institut Pasteur* **12** 225.

11) Keen W (1914) *Animal Experimentation and Medical Progress*. Boston: Houghton Mifflin.

12) Bazy M (1914) *Comp Rendus Soc Biol* **159** 794.

13) Brown A et al. (1960) Value of a large dose of antitoxin in clinical tetanus. *The Lancet* **ii** 227.

14) Sherrington CS (1917) Observations with antithetanus serum in the monkey. *The Lancet* **ii** 964-66.

15) Annotation. *The Lancet* **ii** 464, 1980.

16) Descombey P (1924) L'anatoxine tétanique. *Comp Rendus Soc Biol* **91** 239.

17) Bergey DH & Etris S (1933) Tetanus toxoid in prophylaxis against tetanus. *J Infect Dis* **53** 331. http://dx.doi.org/10.1093/infdis/53.3.331

18) (1979) WHO expert committee on biological standardization. Thirtieth report, technical report series 638 World Health Organization, Geneva. http://dx.doi.org/10.1016/0016-6480(80)90066-0

19) Long A & Sartwell P (1947) Tetanus in the United States Army in World War II. *Bull US Army Med Dept* **7** 371.

20) Christenson B & Bottiger M (1987) Epidemiology and immunity to tetanus in Sweden. *Scand J Infect Dis* **19** 429.

21) Simonsen O et al. (1987) Epidemiology of tetanus in Denmark 1920-1982. Ibid. **19** 437.

22) Cryz S (1991) *Vaccines and Immunotherapy*. New York: Pergamon.

23) Habig W & Tankersley D (1991) (in Cryz above).

24) Newell K et al. (1966) The use of toxoid for the prevention of tetanus neonatorum. Final report of a double-blind controlled field trial. *Bull WHO* **35** 863.

25) Smith J & Collee J (1990) Tetanus, in *Topley & Wilson's Principles of Bacteriology, Virology & Immunity*, vol. 3. London: Edward Arnold.

26) Schiavo G et al. (1992) Tetanus and botulinum-B neurotoxins block neurotransmitter release by proteolytic cleavage of synaptobrevin. *Nature* **359** 832.

27) *The Independent* 10 August 1993.

(1991) *Index of Veterinary Specialities* **31** no 1.

4. Pertussis Vaccine, Unfairly Maligned – At What Cost?

Whooping cough prophylaxis, as pertussis vaccine, is routinely administered to infants together with diphtheria and tetanus as the DPT combined immunisation.

After a short catarrhal phase, whooping cough begins with a dry nocturnal cough. This progresses to prolonged bouts of coughing which often end with a sharp intake of breath. The coughing fits may induce vomiting and, in severe cases, convulsions. Frank damage to the nervous system may occur, this is due to haemorrhage and lack of oxygen in the brain caused by the raised venous pressure that occurs during the paroxysms.

The symptoms persist for weeks and may be complicated by pneumonia, bronchitis and collapse of the lung. Admission to intensive care is frequently required. The patient may be left in a debilitated condition with an increased susceptibility to pulmonary infections. Whooping cough is without doubt an extremely distressing disease for both the patients and carers.

Prior to vaccination, mortality to whooping cough was the highest for any childhood disease. In Europe and the USA between 1900 and the 1920s the annual death rate was between 10 and 11 per 100,000 (mostly children under 3 years). In 1931, a standard textbook of bacteriology stated: "[whooping cough] may be looked upon as one of the major causes of death in civilised countries." At this time it was responsible for 1.3% of all deaths in England and Wales (1). Today, whooping cough is still a significant cause of child mortality in developing countries. In 1991 it was estimated that, world-wide, pertussis caused the deaths of approximately 340,000 children each year (25).

The causative organism of whooping cough was described in 1900 when Bordet and Gengou observed small, ovoid bodies in the sputum of a child

http://dx.doi.org/10.11647/OBP.0055.04

with the disease. Cultivation of the bacillus (*Bordetella pertussis*) was not achieved until 1906 when the same workers managed to grow the organism on a composite medium of glycerin extract of potato, agar and defibrinated rabbit blood (2).

Toxins obtained from these cultures were lethal to rabbits after intravenous injection. Subcutaneous injection produced a non-suppurating local necrosis (1). The pathological effects in humans are presumably due to local necrosis caused by toxins released by the bacilli growing on the ciliated cells lining the bronchi and trachea. A thick, ropy exudate is formed and the attempted ejection of this, together with a systemic effect of pertussis toxin, is the cause of the paroxysmal cough.

The Vaccine

It was natural that researchers should attempt to develop a vaccine that would protect against such a distressing disease with a high child mortality. Clinical trials began in the 1920s to determine the protective effect conferred by extracts of killed *Bordetella pertussis*. The vaccines were generally considered to confer some degree of protection, although the studies were not always well-controlled (3).

To assess the potential of the various vaccines against whooping cough, a series of rigorous trials under the control of the Medical Research Council began in England after World War II and were completed in 1959. This whole investigation was of impeccable quality and reflected great credit on the relevant committee of the MRC.

It soon became apparent that the candidate vaccines varied in ability to protect against the disease. It was thus decided to assess the correlation between the efficacy of the vaccines in children and the potency in the "mouse protection test." In this test, groups of 15 mice were injected with graded doses of vaccine, and 10-14 days later challenged intracerebrally with a virulent strain of the bacillus. From the proportion of mice dying in each group an estimate of the efficacy of the vaccine could be obtained. In a study of 25 vaccines there was a high degree of correlation between the activity in the mouse test and the effectiveness of the vaccine in the field (4). These meticulous observations thus provided a quick method of assessment of new vaccine preparations, and the final report of the MRC trials recommended (5): "Only those pertussis vaccines which have been shown, by the intracerebral mouse protection test, to have adequate potency in relation to the British Standard Pertussis Vaccine should be used in whooping cough prophylaxis."

The MRC trials, double-blind and randomised as they were, showed definitively that vaccination against pertussis was effective. Immunisation of infants was therefore officially recommended in 1957, although immunisation had already spread throughout some areas of England and Wales during the 1940s and early 1950s as local health authorities gradually adopted a pertussis immunisation programme and replaced diphtheria/tetanus vaccine with diphtheria/tetanus/pertussis vaccine in their routine procedures (6) (Fig. 4.1).

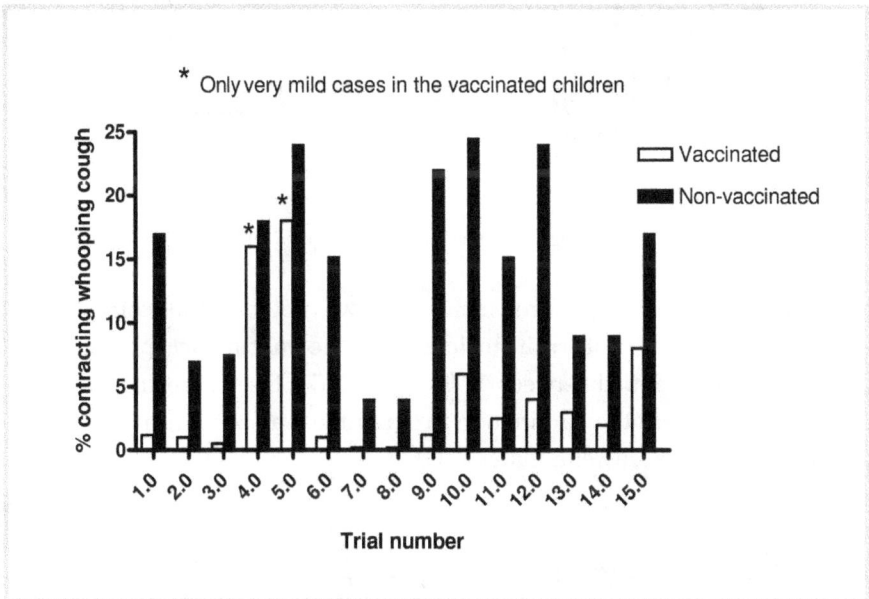

Fig. 4.1 Studies on pertussis immunisation, 1937-1942. 1.0 Saur 1938; 2.0 Park 1937; 3.0 Kendrick Eldering 1939; 4.0 Doull-Shipley 1939; 5.0 Kramer 1938; 6.0 Silverthorne 1939; 7.0 Siegel 1938; 8.0 Siegel 1938; 9.0 Singer 1940; 10.0 Howell 1938; 11.0 Kendrick Eldering 1939; 12.0 Kositza 1940; 13.0 Lapin et al 1939; 14.0 Lapin et al 1939; 15.0 Perkins 1942.[1]

The beneficial effect of routine vaccination against whooping cough is well illustrated by the drop in incidence in England and Wales as the vaccination acceptance rate rose to around 80% (Fig. 4.2).

---

1   Data taken from J H Lapin (1943) *Whooping Cough*. London: CC Thomas, from which complete references may be obtained.

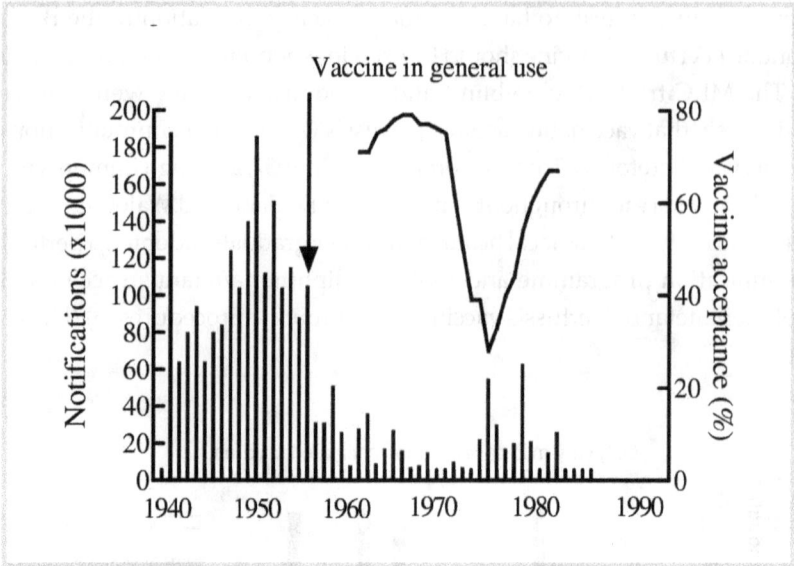

Caption: Fig. 4.2 Whooping cough notifications in England and Wales, 1940-1990.

Clear confirmation that the drop in incidence was not fortuitous coincidence is provided by the upturn in incidence as the vaccine acceptance rate unfortunately dropped between 1975 and 1983 (7). Elsewhere, in countries such as Fiji, where the vaccination programme was not interrupted, the disease was practically eliminated (8) (Fig. 4.3).

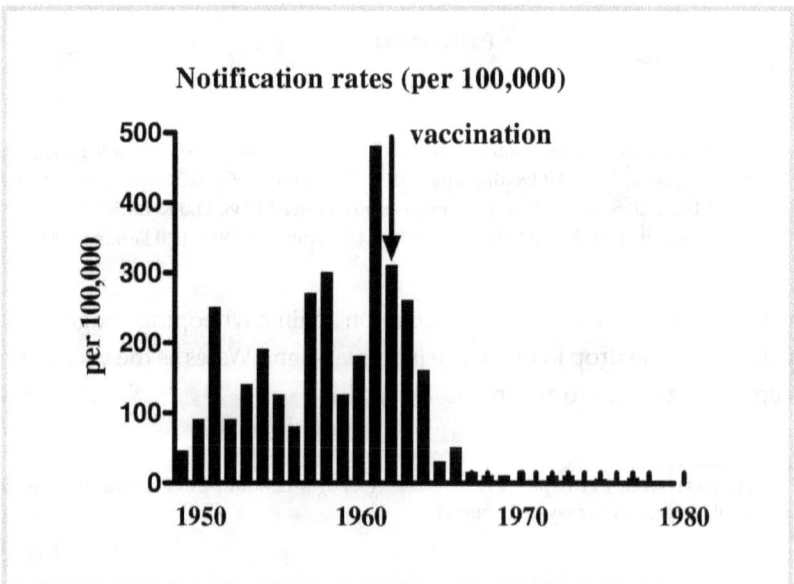

Fig. 4.3 Whooping cough in Fiji, 1950-1980.

Questions of Safety

Undoubtedly, the killed, whole cell pertussis vaccine is highly reactogenic. Redness and soreness at the site of injection and fever are common. Incidence of serious reactions such as persistent screaming, convulsions or shock accompanied by collapse have been variously estimated as 1 in 5000 to 1 in 50,000 injections (9), although these studies were never controlled and thus neglected the natural incidence of these events. For example, a first convulsion may occur naturally in approximately 1 child in 400 aged between 3-9 months. Thus one child in 10,000 in that age group, given 3 doses of vaccine might by chance have a first convulsion within 3 days of an injection (7).

The great contention that has dogged discussion of the safety of pertussis vaccine for the last two decades is whether it occasionally produces irreversible brain damage. The history of the rise and fall of this canard should be mandatory study for both medical students and science writers.

There were sporadic reports of an alleged association between pertussis vaccination and serious brain damage but these were paid little heed since control studies were never performed and most informed authorities did not assume a causal relationship (9). The discussion was kept within the medical establishment and thus did not affect the acceptance rate of pertussis vaccination by the public.

A crucial event was the publication in 1974 of a paper that stated that over an 11 year period, 36 children were admitted to a large London hospital with acute neurological illness that had started within 28 days of an injection of pertussis vaccine (10). The authors made no claim that the vaccination caused the illness and in some of the cases there were probable diagnoses that excluded an assumption of a causal relationship. This report might well have remained accessible only to those capable of assessing the significance of these observations in conjunction with other valuable epidemiological studies. Unfortunately the mass media gave them much publicity with the result that the general public and some general practitioners (but not consultant paediatricians) were reluctant to accept pertussis immunisation.

Between 1977 and 1983 the question of whether or not pertussis vaccine caused irreversible brain damage continued to be argued. On one side allegations of an incidence of 1 in 60,000 to 1 in 10,000 were quoted (11); on the other the possibility was described as "not proven" or very rare (1 in 135,000 to 1 in 300,000) (12, 24). The problem was the temptation (to some) to accept that any neurological defect that developed after vaccination was necessarily caused by it. Natural incidences of neurological problems in infants were ignored. The diagnostic problems of assigning a severe encephalopathy to vaccination were well illustrated by the clinical account of 3 children who developed mental handicap, symptoms of which appeared 6 hours, 2 days and 1 week respectively after "the whooping cough jab" (12). These children might well have remained designated as "vaccine damaged" but for follow up studies one and a half to four years later, which showed two of the children had suffered prenatal damage and the third had X-linked Menkes disease inherited from his maternal grandmother. In the same paper the pertinent point was made that if, as some suggested, 1:20,000 children vaccinated with pertussis suffered brain damage, then there should be enough affected children for each specialist in paediatric neurology to have an appreciable case load of children with a characteristic disease indubitably associated with vaccination. This was not the case.

The relative danger of forgoing vaccination for a perceived risk of, say a 1 in 135,000 chance of serious neurological damage, were well illustrated by Grist in 1977 (13). He claimed that 135,000 cases of whooping cough "would entail 30 cases of encephalitis..., many cases of convulsions, 170 deaths and 13,500 illnesses requiring hospital admission; many children would have pneumonia, bronchitis, and lung damage, and most of them would experience distressing symptoms for many weeks."

The safety of pertussis vaccine has now been established following the comprehensive survey by Pollock and Morris (14) which found no evidence that DPT caused major neurological damage. This has been confirmed by two recent large scale studies from Britain (15) and the USA (16). The first concludes "(the) study has clearly shown that illnesses leading to death or brain damage after diphtheria, tetanus, and pertussis vaccine, if they occur at all, are extremely rare." The second, which involved 218,000 children, "did not find any statistically significant increased risk of onset of serious acute neurological illness in the 7 days after DTP vaccine exposure for young children."

The reassurance provided by these thorough studies comes years too late for the 102,000 children who became seriously ill (32 died) in the epidemic of 1977-79, which coincided with the dramatic decline in vaccine acceptance due to misplaced publicity of brain damage incorrectly attributed to the vaccine. As others have noted with some cynicism (17, 18), the good news of the establishment of the safety of pertussis vaccine has apparently gone unnoticed by the media. Fortunately, the information was actively promoted by the Department of Health with the result that confidence in the vaccine returned and the acceptance rate has risen to 92%.

The Antivivisection Argument

The heated epidemiological arguments over the safety of pertussis that waged for 10-15 years provided an opportunity for the promulgation of persuasive propaganda by those opposed to animal experiments. Sharpe, for example (21), quotes only data from Stewart, who was virtually the sole advocate of the rejection of the vaccine on grounds of safety. This view was emphatically but courteously attacked in the medical journals by both neurologists and paediatricians (12, 13, 19, 20). This contention was quite overt and was not only carried out in the correspondence columns of the *British Medical Journal* and the *Lancet*, but also featured in editorials and leading articles. These discussions are ignored by Sharpe, as is the substantial study by Pollock and Morris (14) (which absolves the vaccine) and the scholarly and well-balanced review by Miller, Alderslade and Ross (9), both of which appeared 5 years before the publication of Sharpe's attack on animal experimentation, *The Cruel Deception*. The misrepresentation that results from selection of evidence solely supporting one's prejudice is in itself a deception.

Sharpe also questions the benefit produced by pertussis vaccination. He presents a graph (with no scale or actual figures) which shows a steep fall in mortality due to whooping cough from 1860 onwards (23). He thus claims that the disease had ceased to be a problem before the advent of antibiotics or vaccination. Mortality certainly had fallen due to great improvements in the techniques applied to the care of infants with respiratory disease. Application of specialist nursing, techniques of aspiration, the availability of intensive care units, oxygen etc., all contributed, as did the availability of antibiotics to combat secondary infections. Nonetheless to suggest that the disease was of little significance is a travesty.

The incidence of the disease did not diminish until vaccination. Even if mortality was reduced, whooping cough was a severe and dangerous disease in a substantial proportion of affected children, as the epidemic of 1977-79 showed. The problem was well illustrated by the Royal College of General Practitioners special report on the nature of this epidemic in a large population of West Glamorgan (22). 2,295 cases were reported, two children died of apparent cot death, 64 unvaccinated children had to be admitted to hospital, 24 needed aspiration, 25 intensive care, 10 required oxygen. Two had encephalitis (one died), 14 had convulsions, 224 had acute bronchitis, 8 had collapsed lung, 17 developed asthma; there were 26 cases of apnoea. Whooping was present in 45% of cases, the paroxysms were followed by vomiting in 66%. Severe cyanosis after paroxysms occurred in 430 cases. The avoidance of morbidity and mortality of this magnitude would appear a sound justification for the adoption of pertussis immunisation.

The Future

The anxiety over the possible severe adverse effects of the whole cell pertussis vaccine, needless as it was, nevertheless reduced public confidence in the vaccination programme. It is thus important to restore this confidence by the development of a vaccine which contains the antigenic fractions, and no active pertussis toxin or extraneous matter that is likely to cause the local reactions and fever.

A number of candidate vaccines have been produced based on antigenic fractions of precipitates of centrifuged suspensions of bacteria (23). The possible value of these vaccines can be rapidly assessed by their ability to protect mice against intranasal challenge with B pertussis or direct challenge with pertussis toxin. The possibility of reversion to frank toxicity, which has been observed with some potential pertussis vaccines, can be excluded by two simple tests in mice; the histamine sensitisation test or the measurement of leukocytosis-promoting activity (23). An *in vitro* test is now available for pertussis toxin based on the morphological changes it produces in Chinese hamster ovary cells.

An earlier version of this chapter was published as: Pertussis vaccine, unfairly maligned – at what cost? *RDS News* April 1994 10-13.

References

1) Zinssner H (1931) *Textbook of Bacteriology*. 6th ed. New York: Appleton.

2) Bordet & Gengou (1906) Le microbe de la coqueluche. *Ann de l'Inst Pasteur* **20** 731.

3) Lapin J (1943) *Whooping Cough*. Springfield: C C Thomas.

4) Medical Research Council (1956) Vaccination against whooping cough. Relation between protection in children and results of laboratory tests. *Br Med J* ii, 454

5) Medical Research Council (1959) Vaccination against whooping cough. Final report. *Br Med J* i, 454-62. http://www.ncbi.nlm.nih.gov/pmc/articles/PMC2034830/

6) Griffith A (1982) ABC of 1 to 7: whooping cough (Letter). *Br Med J* **284** 1263-64.

7) Parker M & Collier L (1990) Topley & Wilson's *Principles of Bacteriology, Virology and Immunity: Systematic Bacteriology*. 8th Edition Volume 3. Hodder Arnold.

8) Pollard R (1983) Whooping cough in Fiji. *The Lancet* i 1381.

9) Miller D, Alderslade R & Ross E (1982) Whooping cough and whooping cough vaccine. The risks and benefits debate. *Epidemiol Rev* **4** 1.

10) Kulenkampff M, Schwartzman J & Wilson J (1974) Neurological complications of pertussis inoculation. *Arch Dis Child* **49** 46.

11) Stewart G (1977) Vaccination against Whooping-cough. Efficacy Versus Risks. *The Lancet* i 234.

12) Stephenson J (1977) Vaccination against whooping-cough. *The Lancet* i 357.

13) Grist G (1977) Vaccination against whooping-cough. *The Lancet* i 358.

14) Pollock T and Morris J (1983) A 7-year Survey of disorders attributed to vaccination in north west Thames Region. *The Lancet* i 753.

15) Miller D et al. (1993) Pertussis immunisation and serious neurological illness in children. *Br Med J* **307** 1171.

16) Gale J et al. (1994) Risk of Serious Acute Neurological Illness after Immunisation with DPT Vaccine. *JAMA* **271** 1.

17) Paton W (1993) *Man and Mouse: Animals in Medical Research*. Oxford: Oxford University Press.

18) Minerva Med (1983) Views. *Br Med J* **286** 1288, http://www.ncbi.nlm.nih.gov/pmc/articles/PMC1547286/?page=1

19) Miller D and Ross E (1982) ABC of 1 to 7: Whooping cough. *Br Med J* **284** 1874.

20) Preston N (1982) Toxicity of pertussis vaccine. *Br Med J* **284** 1817.

21) Sharpe R (1988) *The Cruel Deception: The Use of Animals in Medical Research*. London: Thorsons.

22) Royal College of General Practitioners (1981) Report from the Swansea Research Unit. Effect of a low pertussis vaccination uptake on a large community. *Br Med J* **282** 23. http://www.ncbi.nlm.nih.gov/pmc/articles/PMC1503761/

23) Cryz S (1991) *Vaccines and Immunotherapy*. New York: Pergamon.

24) Valman H (1982) Whooping cough. *Br Med J* **284** 886.

25) Galazka A (1992) Control of pertussis in the world. *Wld Hlth Statist Quart* **45** 886.

5. Vaccination: The Present and Future

Meningitis

The reduction of morbidity and mortality through development of new or improved vaccines continues. In October 1992, vaccination against infection by *Haemophilus influenzae* type B (Hib), a major cause of meningitis, was included in the childhood immunisation programme in Britain. The effect was immediate, for Hib infections fell by 70% in the period January to March, 1993 (1).

The introduction of the vaccine in Britain was triggered by the outstanding success of the experiment in Finland, where the introduction of the vaccine in 1986 reduced the incidence of Hib menigitis, which had been steadily rising since the 1960s, to zero by 1991 (2) (Fig. 5.1).

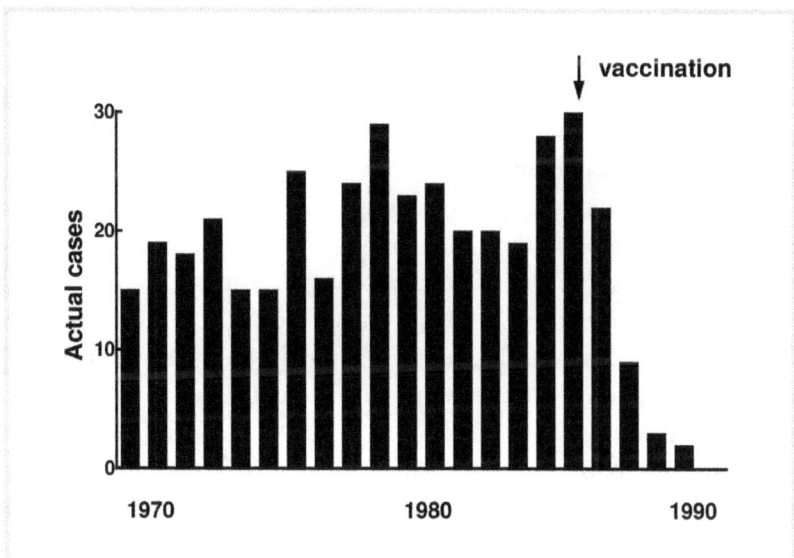

Fig. 5.1 Hib meningitis in Helsinki. Actual cases, 1970-1990.

http://dx.doi.org/10.11647/OBP.0055.05

Similar benefit had been reported in three regional studies of Hib meningitis in the USA, where falls in incidence of between 80-90% occurred over a two year period following vaccination against Hib (3) (Fig. 5.2).

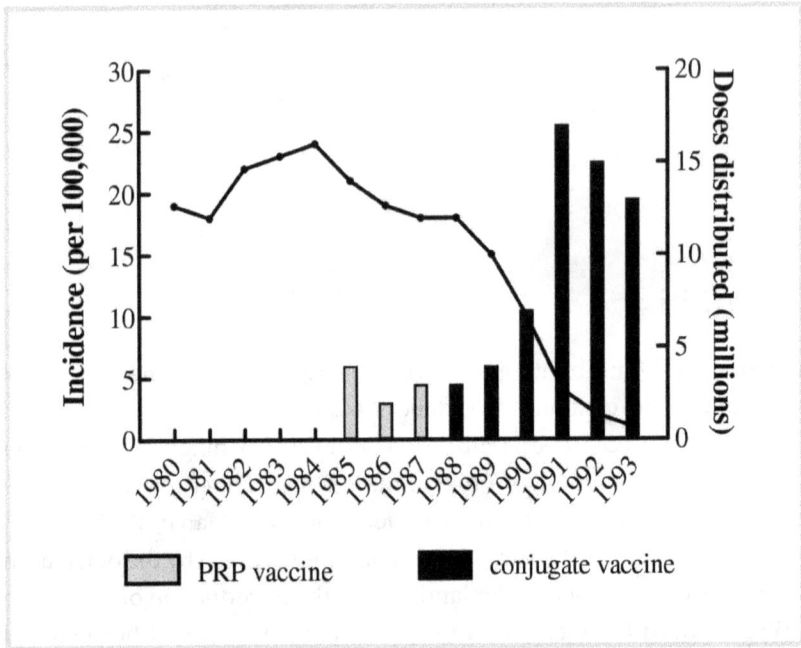

Fig. 5.2 Decline of Hib Meningitis in USA children under 5 years, 1980-1993.

Prior to vaccination, 1500 cases of Hib infection occurred every year in the UK (mostly in children under one year), over half resulting in meningitis. Despite the effectiveness of antibiotics against the bacillus, it killed 65 children and caused permanent brain damage, deafness etc. in a further 150 each year.

The drive to produce a prophylaxis against this potentially devastating disease was considerable, but initial efforts were stymied by the nature of the antigen. This is a polysaccharide present in the capsule of the bacterium, a linear polymer of ribose, ribitol and phosphate (PRP). Antibodies to PRP were effective at passively immunising animals, but PRP vaccines could only produce a poor, short-lived immunity in children under one year, that is those at greatest risk.

After much experimentation the immunogenicity of PRP was increased by coupling it to a protein. This general technique had been suggested by the work of Landsteiner (of blood group fame) and had been shown to be effective in protecting mice against infection with pneumococci (4). Conjugates of PRP with bovine or human albumin, haemocyanin and diphtheria toxoid were shown to be powerfully immunogenic in mice and rabbits (4). From these experimental studies four effective vaccines were developed for human use, based on PRP linked to diphtheria toxoid, tetanus toxoid or a membrane protein from meningococci. Each vaccine was of course subject to the standard animal tests for innocuity.

Malaria

In terms of extent, malaria is one of the most serious infectious diseases. Actual numbers of those affected are difficult to establish, due to the remoteness of some of the areas where the disease is endemic. A recent estimate suggested that malaria causes 3 million deaths per year in Africa alone, one third of these being children under 5 years of age (5). The parasite is generally developing resistance to antimalarial drugs, as is the anopheles mosquito to insecticides. An effective vaccine has thus long been sought and may now have been found since the prototype vaccine SPf66 has been shown to produce a "strong immune response" in a recent trial in Tanzania (5). SPf66, developed by Patarroyo at the University of Bogota, was perfected by experiments in aotus monkeys (6).

The Future

What next? Will research to produce new vaccines become redundant? Hardly. The spectre of AIDS still looms, other fatal diseases emerge and old diseases re-emerge as problems.

Tuberculosis is on the increase in certain areas and paediatricians are questioning the policy of some health authorities to discontinue routine BCG vaccinations, this despite the advice of the British Thoracic Society to continue to offer BCG to all 10 to 14-year-olds and neonates in areas where the incidence of tuberculosis is high (7).

An emergent problem is posed by hantaviruses. An estimated 200,000 people world-wide become infected with hantaviruses each year, between 4,000 and 20,000 die as a result (8). Hantaviruses, which produce haemorrhagic fever and chronic nephropathy, normally infect rodents, but can easily spread to humans under certain conditions. In October 1993, the US Center for Disease Control and Prevention confirmed that there were 42 cases (with

26 deaths) of a new disease, hantavirus pulmonary syndrome. This had presumably arisen due to the sudden proliferation of the rodent population in SW states caused by unusual social and climatic changes (9). Hantavirus infections are virtually untreatable. The development of a vaccine is the only way to combat the threat of an epidemic.

The denial of the importance of animals in research into the nature and treatment of infective disease, and the insistence of animal rights groups that economic and social change is the sole cause of the decrease in morbidity and death from infection cannot be sustained. The consequent questioning of the effectiveness of vaccination, and the promulgation of unsupportable allegations of the toxicity of vaccines, is at best unjustified and in some instances thoroughly irresponsible (see for example 10).

VACCINES INTRODUCED FOR HUMAN USE.
From Cryz SJ (1991) *Vaccines and Immunotherapy.* New York: Pergamon.

1880	Rabies
1890	Typhoid, cholera, plague
1920	Diphtheria, pertussis, tetanus,tuberculosis
1930	Yellow fever, scrub typhus
1940	Influenza, pneumococcal pneumonia
1950	Poliomyelitis
1960	Measels, mumps, rubella
1970	Meningococcal meningitis
1980	Adenovirus, Hepatitis B, Hib meningitis

An earlier version of this chapter was published as: Vaccination: the present and future. *RDS News* April 1994 14-15.

References

1) Anon (1993) Fall in childhood Hib infection reported. *Pharm J* **250** 633.

2) Peltola H, Kilpi T, Anttila M (1992) Rapid disappearance of haemophilus influenzae type B meningitis after routine childhood immunisation with conjugate vaccines. *The Lancet* **340** 592

3) Dixon B (1993) Microbe of the month. *The Independent*, February 8.

4) Sood S & Daum R (1991) in *Vaccines and Immunotherapy*. ed Cryz S. New York: Pergamon.

5) *The Independent*, February 14 1994.

6) News and political reviews. *Br Med J* (1991) **302** 432.

7) Anon (1993) Fall in childhood Hib infection in USA. *Pharm J* **251** 216.

8) Dixon B (1993) Microbe of the month. *The Independent*, December 13.

9) Levins R et al. (1993) Hantavirus disease emerging. *The Lancet* **342** 1292.

10) Williams L (1993) A shot in the dark. *The Guardian* July 20.

6. The Conquest of Polio and the Contribution of Animal Experiments

Any individual old enough to have even occasional recall of a childhood before World War II must be aware of the impact of antibacterial agents and vaccination on infective disease.

With the advent of prontosil and hence the sulphonamides, followed by the antibiotics, death from common bacterial infections has become a comparative rarity. Similarly, the leg braces and iron lungs (Fig. 6.1) – a mark of the epidemics of poliomyelitis that were a regular feature of Europe and North America throughout the first half of the twentieth century – are now seen only in the countries which have not yet implemented the polio vaccination programme instituted by the WHO.

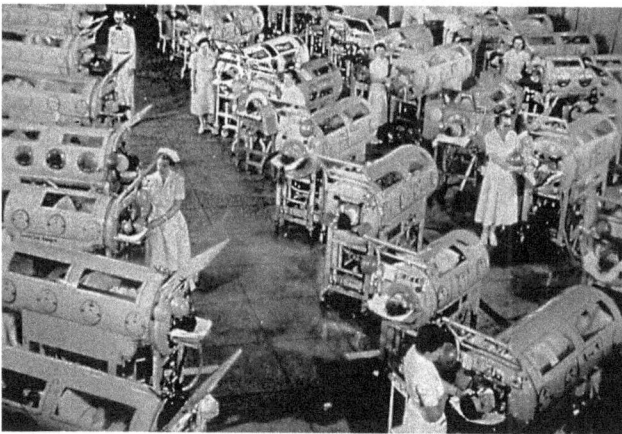

Fig. 6.1 The iron lung before vaccination, 1952? Image in the public domain.

http://dx.doi.org/10.11647/OBP.0055.06

Those who assert that animal experiments have contributed nothing to the treatment of infectious disease claim that improvements in hygiene and sanitation are solely responsible for the lower death and morbidity from infectious disease this century.

It is undoubtedly true that improvements in social conditions lessen the possibility of contraction of certain bacterial diseases, and that improvements in nutrition may increase resistance. It is, however, undeniable that the annual death rate from puerperal sepsis was steady at approximately 190/100,000 births from 1860 to 1938, but with the development of sulphonamides and antibiotics this had fallen to half that value within two years, and to approximately 5/100,000 by the 1960s (1).

Similarly, the death rate from lobar pneumonia in middle-aged men averaged a steady 60/100,000 from 1910-1940, but with the application of bacterial chemotherapy had fallen to below 6 by 1970 (2).

However, of all the contentions of the animal rights movement, its attempts to reject the contribution of animal experiments towards the reduction in death and paralysis from poliomyelitis are the most unacceptable. Thus it is claimed:

> The significance of poliomyelitis had dropped as better sanitation, better housing, cleaner water and better food had been introduced in the second half of the 19th century. (3)

This statement is quite untrue. For 4,000 years 'infantile paralysis' was a sporadic disease, with a very low background occurrence. A dramatic change occurred at the end of the nineteenth century, when epidemics began to occur in Scandinavia (1868-1881) and later in Vermont, USA (1894). The 1905 epidemic in Sweden (1031 cases) established the change in nature of the condition from an obscure, endemic, sporadic disease to one with a regular, almost predictable occurrence in *developed* countries (4) (Fig. 6.2).

What explanation can account for this apparent paradox, that poliomyelitis only became a serious problem in those countries (e.g. in late nineteenth century Scandinavia) that boasted the *highest* standards of hygiene and sanitation? In fact poliomyelitis can be relatively innocuous if contracted when one is very young. Symptoms may be confined to a temperature and headache – a so-called "inapparent infection" – yet this can confer life-long immunity. It is thus obvious that infants brought up in unsanitary conditions are likely to become infected whilst very young, suffer a slight illness and become immune. As hygiene and sanitation improve children become shielded from infection during infancy, and thus may contract the condition at an age when they are particularly vulnerable to the severe, paralytic form of the disease. The infection can then easily spread among such non-immune persons and the epidemics, typical of the first half of the 20th century, will result (4).

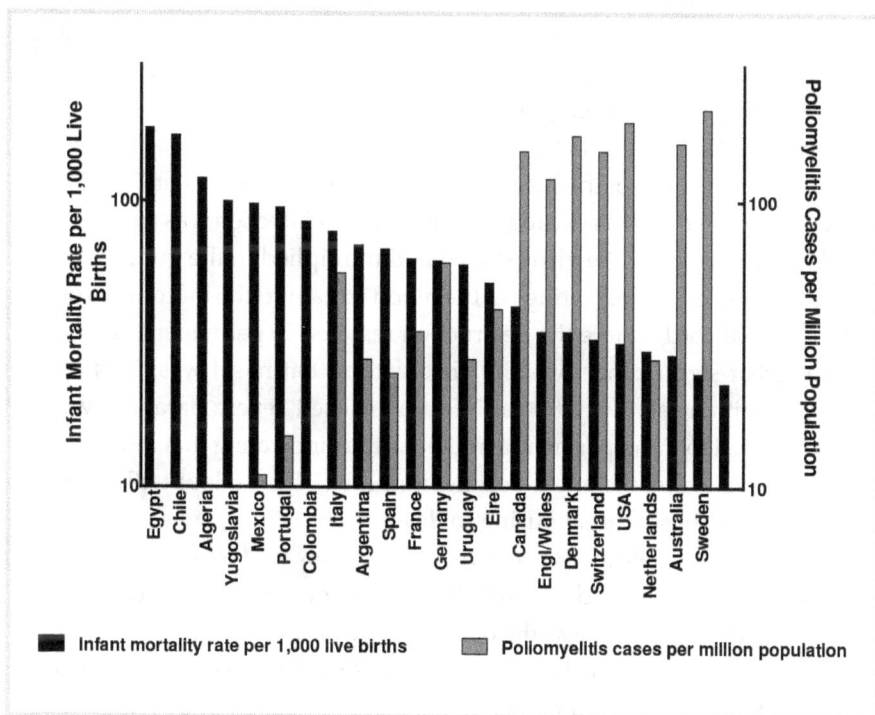

Fig. 6.2 Comparison of infant mortality rates and the incidence of poliomyelitis.

Animal experiments, of course, were crucial in the elucidation of the nature of poliomyelitis and inevitably in the formation of a vaccine. Although it was suspected that polio was an infectious disease, definitive proof was provided in 1908, when Landsteiner and Popper (5) managed to induce the condition in monkeys by injecting homogenates of the spinal cord of a 9-year-old boy who had died of acute polio. Since the samples of spinal cord were shown to be free of bacteria, Landsteiner and Popper surmised that poliomyelitis was caused by a virus too small to be detected by microscopic techniques at that time (in actual fact poliovirus is one of the smallest viruses). The infection was transferred from monkey to monkey and thus provided a model of the disease from which much information was gleaned.

It is unfortunate that Landsteiner, at that time working in Vienna, was not able to continue in this field, since the enormous expense of maintaining a sufficient monkey colony to pursue this study was beyond his available funds. (Landsteiner was awarded the Nobel Prize in 1930 for his work on the classification of blood groups).

From 1908 until the 1940s the induction of polio in monkeys was the only means of study of the disease. With this model it was established that three strains of the virus existed, that the route of infection was *via* the nose and mouth, and that the virus stayed and multiplied in the gut before, in more serious cases, migrating *via* the blood stream to the motor neurones of the spinal cord, where the destruction resulted in permanent paralysis.

Of great significance was the observation that nasal washings from patients with a relatively trivial infection caused severe paralysis when administered to the experimental monkey, thus indicating that individuals *could*, in some circumstances become immune. This undoubtedly served to encourage those endeavouring to develop a vaccine.

From an early date attempts were made to grow the virus in culture, just as bacteria were cultured in broth. Viruses of course can only replicate in cells, thus tissue culture was the only possible means of fostering the virus outside the whole animal. Progress was slow since there were few groups of workers who could afford to maintain a monkey colony. The problem was eased when, after much effort, a strain of poliovirus was transferred to the Cotton rat, and subsequently to the mouse. The maintenance of the poliovirus in mice was significant because it meant that it was now possible to use a sufficient number of animals to provide clear evidence for the existence and virulence of the poliovirus. Thus the way was paved for intensive efforts to grow the virus in culture. As animal rights literature claims:

[...] the most crucial breakthrough in preparing the vaccine came in 1949 when Enders and his colleagues showed how poliovirus could be grown in human tissue culture. (6),

and

animal research supporters are wrong to say that without animal experiments there would never have been a vaccine against poliomyelitis because: an early breakthrough in the development of poliomyelitis vaccine was made in 1949 with the aid of a human tissue culture. (3)

It is certainly true that Enders and his co-workers (7) made a significant advance in showing that the poliovirus could be grown in culture and for this they were awarded the Nobel Prize in 1954. However, for animal rights groups to imply that this work was a significant departure from animal experimentation is absolutely wrong. Further it has to be said that anyone who implies as such (if they have any scientific pretensions) are either deluding themselves or deliberately attempting to mislead the general public.

The poliovirus could not be seen, how was it therefore possible to establish that the virus was replicating in culture? Only by an animal experiment. The primary inoculum seeded by Enders was a suspension of brain tissue from a mouse that had been infected with the Lansing strain of poliovirus. (The identity of the virus was verified by the *"character of the disease it produced in white mice following intracerebral injection"*). Subcultures to fresh tissue were prepared at 8-20 day intervals. Replication of the virus was proven when at the end of 67 days culture the primary inoculum had been diluted by many millions. Even so, the culture fluid still: *"on inoculation into mice and monkeys, produced typical paralysis."* Thus, animal experiments were crucial in these significant results. It is probably superfluous to add that the incubation fluid used by Enders et al. was "balanced salt solution (3 parts) and ox serum ultrafiltrate (1 part)."

The ability to grow the virus in cell culture ensured the rapid development of a vaccine, and widespread vaccination was introduced in 1955 in the USA and Europe (Figs. 6.3 and 6.4).

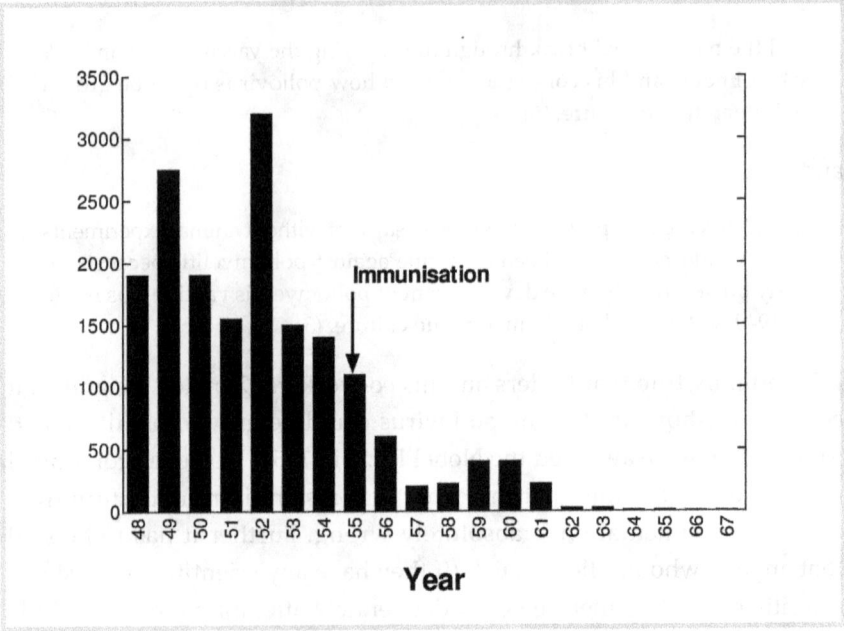

Fig. 6.3 Deaths from poliomyelitis in the USA, 1948-1967. Data from Vital statistics of the USA; US Dept of Health, Educ. & Welfare.

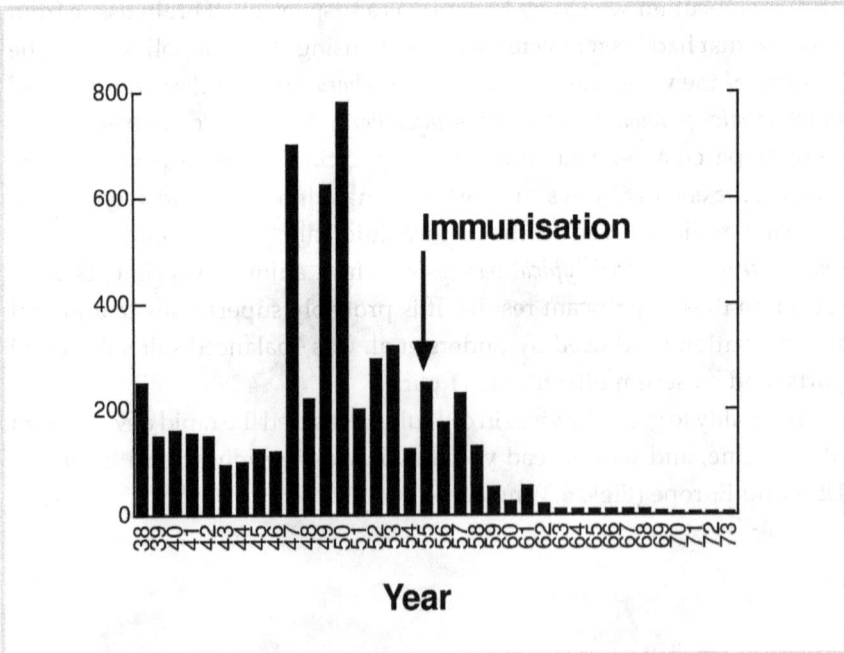

Fig. 6.4 Deaths from poliomyelitis in England and Wales, 1938-1973.
A.M. Ramsey and R.T.D. Emond, *Infectious Diseases*, London: Heinemann, 1978.

As a result, the disease has been virtually eliminated from these areas. It has been estimated that 1.5 million cases of polio were prevented in the decade 1980-1990 due to the immunisation programme (8). Although one opponent of animal experiments claims: "Proof that the introduction of the (polio) vaccine was not the success it was made out to be comes from undeniable statistics" (3), mortality and morbidity figures do not in any way support this. Furthermore, the collective medical experience of the WHO maintains that the vaccination programme would eradicate poliomyelitis by the end of the decade (8) (Fig. 6.5).

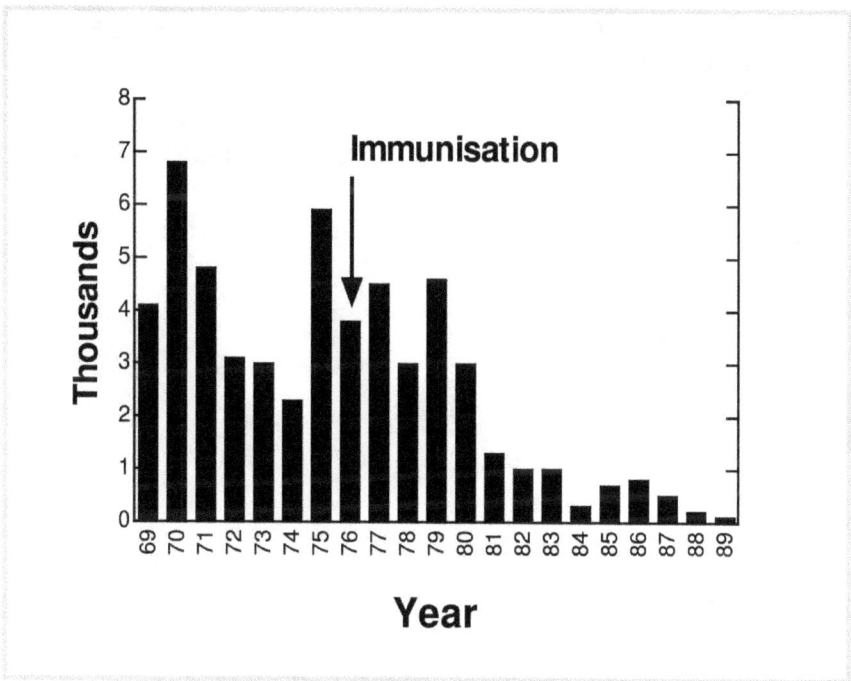

Fig. 6.5 Polio in Latin America, confirmed cases per year, 1969-1989.
Data from *Medical & Health Annual, 1991*, Chicago: Encycl. Britannica Inc.

An earlier version of this chapter was published as: The conquest of polio and the contribution of animal experiments. *RDS News* October 1991 4-5.

References

1) (1966) *Disorders Which Shorten Life* Report No 21. Office of Health Economics, London. https://www.ohe.org/publications/disorders-which-shorten-life

2) Anderson T (1977) The role of medicine. *The Lancet* **i**, 747.

3) Coleman V (1991) *Why Animal Experiments Must Stop.* London: Green Print.

4) Paul J R (1971) *A History of Poliomyelitis.* New Haven: Yale University Press.

5) Landsteiner K & Popper E (1908) Mikroscopische Praparate von einem menschlichen und zwei Affenruckenmarken. *Wien klinWschr*, 21, 1830.

6) Sharpe R (1988) *The Cruel Deception: The use of Animals in Medical Research.* London: Thorsons.

7) Enders J, Weller T & Robbins F (1949) Cultivation of the Lansing Strain of Poliomyelitis Virus in Cultures of Various Human Embryonic Tissues. *Science*, 109, 85.

8) *The State of the World's Children*, UNICEF (1991), Oxford: Oxford University press. http://www.unicef.org/sowc/archive/ENGLISH/The%20State%20of%20 the%20World%27s%20Children%201991.pdf

7. Diphtheria: Understanding, Treatment and Prevention

Diphtheria levies a toll of clinical incidence of 10% of all born with a mortality of 5 to 7 per 1000; immunisation reduces this to an incidence of 1% and zero mortality.

Report of Medical Officers of Health,
Diphtheria Immunisation in Infancy,
The Medical Officer (1932) **48** 188.

In the sanitary 1990s it is hard to envisage the experiences of physicians working in the fever hospitals a century ago. Yet this is the only way to appreciate the progress made in the treatment and prevention of infective disease. An inability, or unwillingness, to undertake this exercise largely explains the misrepresentation by some of the value of early treatments of infections. These treatments stemmed from basic research into causative agents and mechanisms of toxicity.

A prime example is diphtheria. The melancholic effect of having to watch a succession of children die either from suffocation or, as the disease progressed, from paralysis and heart failure, was wretched enough. Add to this the demoralisation and sense of impotence caused by the lack of effective treatment, then one can appreciate how dispiriting the practice of medicine could be at that time.

Diphtheria was formally described by Bretonneau in 1826, although epidemics among children of "malignant sore throat destroying life by suffocation and sometimes leaving paralytic sequelae" had been described

http://dx.doi.org/10.11647/OBP.0055.07

since earliest times. The epidemics tended to be cyclical "often lasting for many years, and followed by intervals of quiescence" (1).

The primary lesion of the disease occurs in the upper respiratory tract. It is a thick, leathery, bluish-white pseudomembrane composed of bacteria, dead cells and fibrin. Should the lesion occur in the laryngeal region, the airway may become occluded and intubation would therefore be necessary.

The emergence of the germ theory triggered the start of the scientific investigation of the aetiology of diphtheria. Klebs in 1883 described a bacillus obtained from the pseudomembranes of diphtheria patients. The straight or slightly curved rods described by Klebs we know today were indeed *Corynebacterium diphtheriae,* although Klebs' study was purely morphological. A year later Loeffler isolated and cultured the bacillus from 13 undisputed cases of diphtheria. When the cultures were inoculated onto injured mucous membranes of various animals, pseudomembranes developed, resembling those in patients. Nevertheless, Loeffler's report was somewhat reserved, since he was unable to explain the systemic symptoms of diphtheria.

In both animals and man infected with the supposed causative organism there are severe systemic disturbances and even organ degeneration, but the bacillus could be found only in the local lesion.

The anomaly was resolved in 1888 by the observation by two of Pasteur's colleagues, Roux and Yersin, that the broth used to grow the cultures of *bacillus diphtheriae* remained toxic for guinea pigs after the bacteria had been removed by filtration. The filtered broth was also shown to be toxic for rabbits, dogs, cats and horses (2). Thus the systemic symptoms of the disease were due to the absorption of a toxin exuded during the growth of the bacilli on the mucous membrane. This observation was very important, since studies on hog cholera in 1885 had demonstrated that administration to an animal of very small concentrations of a bacterial product could eventually produce immunity to that infection. Consequently in 1890, von Behring and Kitasato were able to show that administration of very small amounts of diphtheria toxin to animals resulted in the presence in their plasma of a factor which, when mixed with the toxin, rendered it innocuous to animals (3).

The subsequent observation that this plasma, when actually administered to animals, could protect them from fatal doses of diphtheria toxin paved the way for the use of "diphtheria antitoxin" to treat diphtheric patients. According to most accounts the first clinical use of the antitoxin was in Berlin on Christmas Eve 1891, when von Behring administered it to a seriously ill girl who subsequently recovered (Fig. 7.1).

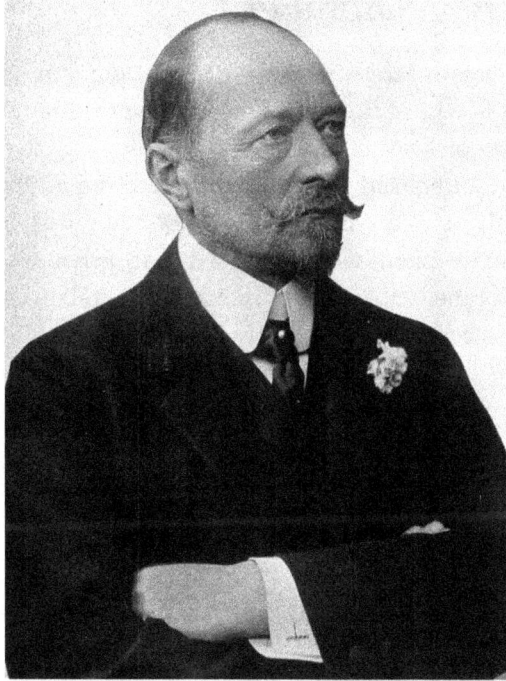

Fig. 7.1 1909 photo of Emil von Behring (1854-1917). Wellcome Library, London, CC BY.

Diphtheria Antitoxin

To produce an effective antitoxin, a potent toxin was required. Typically, a virulent strain of bacillus was grown on a shallow layer of medium and, after 6-8 days, the formed toxin was obtained by filtration. The toxin could only be standardised by a biological assay. This was the measurement of the volume of filtrate that would kill a guinea pig of 250g body weight within 5 days. The lethal volume was required to be below 0.1cc for the toxin to be of adequate strength (4).

The antiserum was usually produced in horses. Gradually increasing subcutaneous doses of toxin were administered over a period of 2-3 months. At the end of this time the horse plasma contained possibly 1,000 antitoxin units per cc and the animal could continue to provide antitoxin for 2-4 years.

The antitoxin in turn required standardisation. This was achieved by comparing its ability to render a sample of toxin innocuous to guinea pigs, with that of a stable, standard sample of antitoxin provided by a central source (4).

Serotherapy in Diphtheria

After the first successful treatment of diphtheria with the antitoxin by von Behring, the use of equine diphtheria antitoxin spread rapidly. Even today serotherapy is the only way to avoid the severe effects of systemic intoxication.

Early on it was realised that to be effective the antitoxin had to be administered early, since the toxin could only be neutralised before it became bound to the tissue elements where it caused toxicity. Rabbits given a tenfold lethal dose of diphtheria toxin could be saved by a relatively small dose of antitoxin if it was administered shortly after the poison. If the injection of the antitoxin was delayed, then increasing doses were required to prevent death. If the administration of the antitoxin occurred after one hour, then no dose would save the animal (4).

Clinical Effects of the Antitoxin

In 1894, Roux and co-workers published their report of the striking benefit produced by antitoxin treatment of diphtheric cases admitted to the Hospital for Sick Children in Paris (5) (Fig. 7.2).

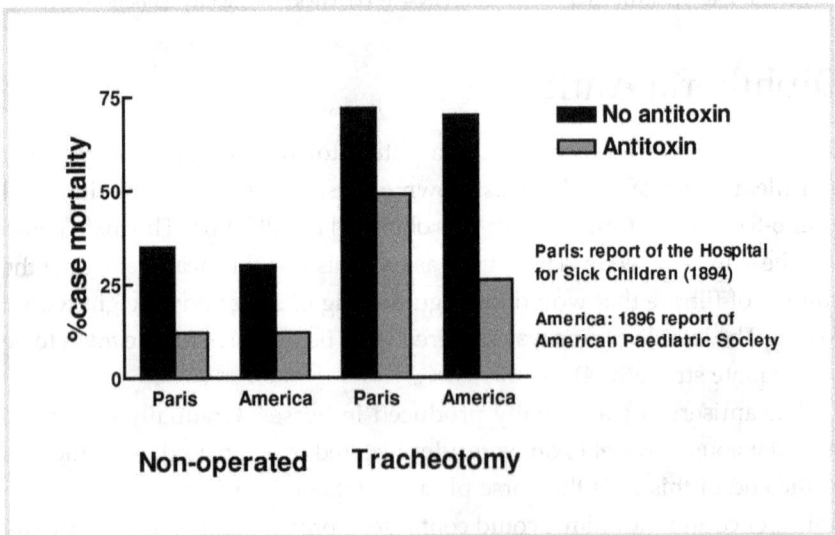

Fig. 7.2 Effect of antitoxin on case mortality.

The serum was administered to every case proved by bacteriological examination to be diphtheric, during February to July 1894. Between 1890-1893, before treatment, 3,971 children were admitted, 2,029 of whom died, a case mortality of

51%. During the first 6 months of serum treatment 448 children were admitted of whom 109 died, a case mortality of 24.3%. During the same period, Trousseau Hospital in Paris was not using the antitoxin, 520 cases were admitted there, 316 died, a case mortality of 60%.

In some cases, where the lesion extended to the laryngeal region, tracheotomy was required. Case mortality in these instances was 73% in the Hospital for Sick Children prior to the use of antiserum. During the trial period this was reduced to 49%, whereas at the Trousseau Hospital the contemporary mortality in such cases was 86%.

After Roux's signal paper, the use of diphtheria antitoxin spread throughout the developed world. Wherever it was used there occurred a reduction in case mortality. Although there was nothing akin to a double-blind clinical trial (case mortalities were compared to those prior to the adoption of the antitoxin) the circumstantial evidence was compelling. Amongst many anecdotes is the oft quoted report of the problem at Baginsky's clinic in Berlin, where they were unfortunate to run out of the antitoxin and the case mortality immediately rose from 15.6% to 48.4% (6).

Based as it was firmly upon experiments in animals, predictably the use of the antiserum came under attack from the antivivisection community. Even as recently as 1934, Beddow Bayly alleged that the antitoxin could not work, since the disease was not caused by the Klebs-Loeffler bacillus but by "drain poison" (7). Strangely, in the same publication he asserts, through selective quotation, that the apparent drop in mortality following the use of antiserum occurred because of diphtheria diagnosis by bacteriological means, i.e. by demonstration of the presence of the bacillus in throat swabs. The result of this was that very mild cases, which previously would have been recorded as minor sore throat, were diagnosed as diphtheria. Beddow Bayly asserted that the inclusion of these mild, self-limiting cases falsely reduced the case mortality. Firstly, this ignores the fact that the reduction in mortality immediately followed the introduction of the antitoxin treatment, whereas the bacillus had been described 10 years previously. Secondly, it takes no heed of the striking reduction in mortality of cases which required tracheotomy, and thus were of undoubted severity. Finally, there were many studies that demonstrated the necessity to administer the antiserum as early as possible, mortality increasing as the treatment was delayed from the first to the fifth day of the disease. As Sir Charles Martin, an authority on the treatment of diphtheria, emphasised: "If the antitoxin were a remedy of no value, whether it were administered on the first or the fifth day of the disease would be immaterial" (8).

Acceptance of the antitoxin was lukewarm in Great Britain. It was not widely used until the publication in 1898 of the report by the Special Committee, set up by the Clinical Society, to investigate the efficacy of antitoxin treatment of diphtheria (9). The report compared 633 treated cases with 3,042 cases that did not receive antitoxin. The 50-page report concluded:

- General mortality is reduced by one-third
- Mortality in tracheotomy falls by one-half
- Extension of the membrane to the larynx very rarely occurs after administration of the antitoxin
- Duration of life in the fatal cases is prolonged
- The number of fatal cases is less when antitoxin is used early in the illness than in those that do not receive it until a later period.

Even after large doses there were no serious ill effects. Rashes occurred in one third of cases. Pain and swelling of the joints were produced in a number of cases.

Immunisation against Diphtheria

As emphasised by Cobbett in 1933 (10), the benefit produced by the antitoxin was "by no means to be despised," but it was only able to reduce the overall case mortality to a certain percentage. This was partly due to the practice of relying on bacteriological diagnosis before administration of the antitoxin, thus delaying the early use of the remedy, when it is most efficacious.

In 1890, von Behring and Kitasato had mooted the possibility of generating active immunity against diphtheria, and had actually produced immunity in guinea pigs by the use of a "detoxified" diphtheria toxin. Some years later, von Behring (11) produced a long-lasting immunity in guinea pigs, monkeys and asses by using a carefully balanced mixture of toxin and antitoxin (a technique which had been used with success in New York for the generation of antitoxin in horses). The toxin/antitoxin mixtures were used in limited studies by von Behring to protect humans against diphtheria, but widespread immunisation only began with the development of formalin-inactivated toxin, introduced independently by Glenny and Hopkins (12) and Ramon (13).

The formalin-inactivated toxoid (and the later alum precipitated and adsorbed diphtheria toxoids) were required to be standardised for antigenic potency by measuring their ability, 28-30 days after inoculation, to protect guinea pigs against a challenge with a 20-fold LD50 of a suitable diphtheria toxin. Innocuity tests also had to be performed to exclude dermal toxicity (intracutaneous injection to rabbits or guinea pigs – observed for 48 hours) and delayed, systemic toxicity (parenteral administration to guinea pigs – observed for 6 weeks) (14).

The adoption of immunisation against diphtheria occurred in piecemeal fashion, its initiation depending on the awareness and energy of individual Medical Officers of Health. There was also a vociferous opposition both from the antivivisection movement and the National Anti-Vaccination League.

From early studies in restricted populations it emerged that sanitary measures of isolation would be of limited value in the containment of diphtheria, since the Health Committee of the League of Nations demonstrated that 97% of infections were not contracted from clinically evident cases of the disease, but from the more numerous healthy carriers of virulent bacilli (8).

The dramatic impact of immunisation was cogently illustrated by the well-controlled investigation of the incidence of cases of diphtheria at Greenwich Hospital School, where immunisation abolished the disease despite the fact that infective but healthy carriers were present in constant numbers both before and after the inoculation programme.

Similarly, striking evidence for the benefits of immunisation against diphtheria comes from the clear protection of nursing and auxiliary staff afforded by inoculation of those deemed to be at risk (i.e. those with a positive Schick test) in diphtheria hospitals (15). Non-immunised staff were 14 times more likely to contract the disease as the inoculated.

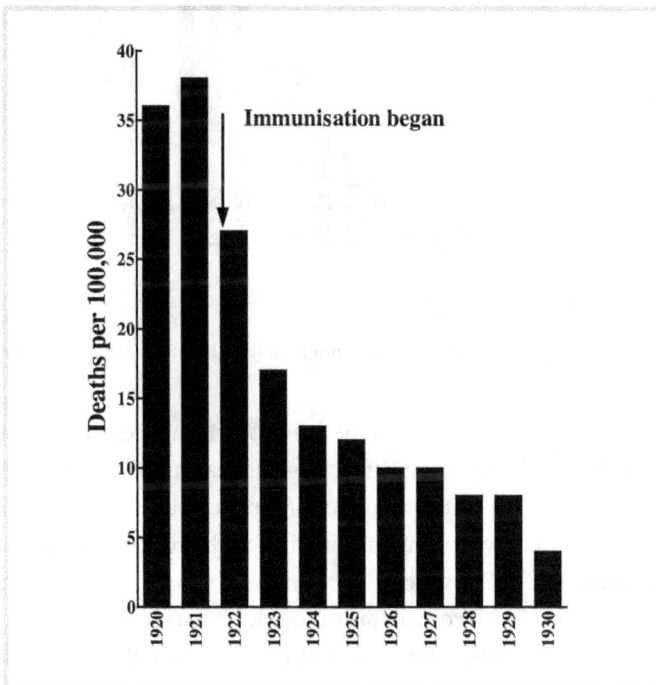

Fig. 7.3 Diphtheria death rate in New York, 1920-1930.

Even in field trials, the benefits of inoculation were clear, for example in New York (described in 1932 as the "best immunised city in the world" (16; Fig. 7.3)) and in Birmingham, which was one of the earliest English cities to institute diphtheria immunisation in 1926. Here a marked decline in incidence of diphtheria was seen by 1931, when almost 10% of children had been vaccinated (17) (Fig. 7.4).

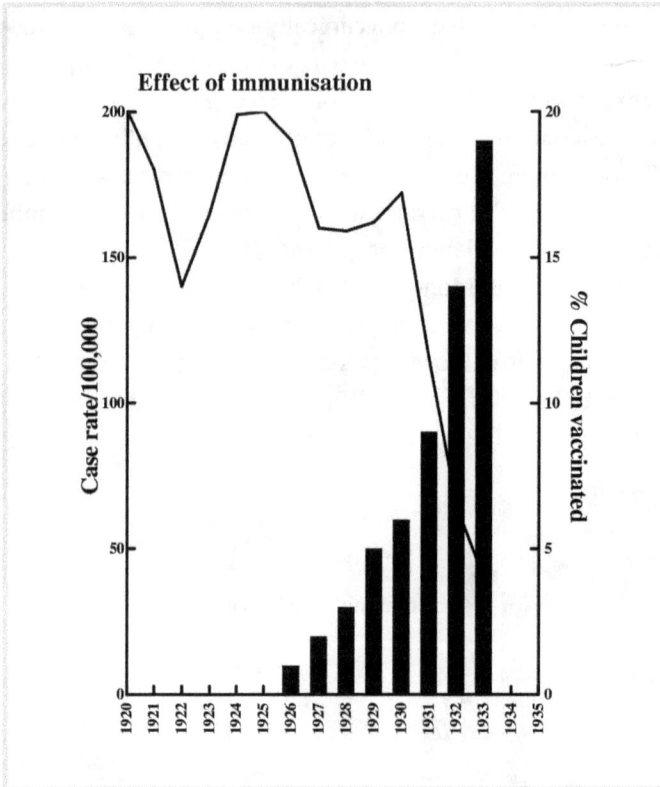

Fig. 7.4 Incidence of diphtheria in Birmingham (children 5-14 years), 1920-1935.

Despite the clear medical evidence of the protection offered by inoculation, the Anti-Vaccination League fought a vigorous rearguard action, disagreeing with immunisation "by filthy concoctions produced from the artificially diseased blood of the lower animals being injected into the clean blood stream of human beings" (18). (The vaccine of course was simply the formalin-treated toxin, it was not obtained from an animal). Much was made of the supposed toxicity of the vaccine (19), although at the time this battle was at its height

(1932), 150,000 persons in Great Britain and Ireland had been immunised against diphtheria without any ill-effect, let alone fatality (20).

The success in local health districts of inoculation against diphtheria resulted in the acceptance across Britain of the immunisation of pre-school children in 1940. The drop in incidence of the disease after this is an impressive illustration of its efficacy (Fig. 7.5).

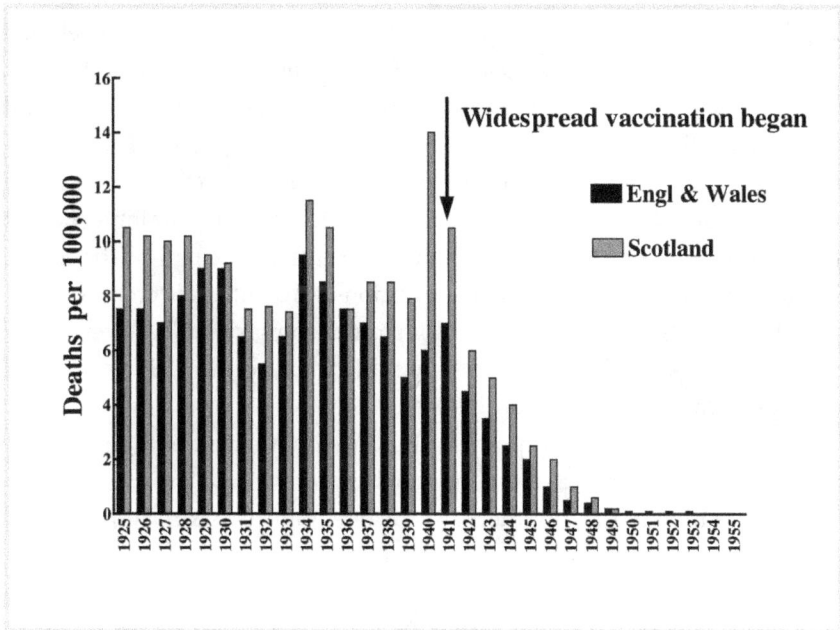

Fig. 7.5 Diphtheria death rate in Great Britain, 1925-1955.

The success of the many local experiments into the protection offered by diphtheria immunisation means there can be no doubt that this technique is effective in reducing the incidence and mortality of the disease. However, as the WHO statistics show (21), in several European countries significant declines in death rates have been registered, despite the fact that in these countries only a few vaccination programmes were carried out in limited areas. It is thus possible that a concurrent change may have taken place in the pathogenicity of *Corynebacterium diphtheriae*, or human resistance may have increased.

It is known that with the increase in the number of resistant individuals as a result of immunisation, the toxinogenic *C diphtheriae* becomes replaced by nontoxinogenic strains in carriers. It is possible this could account for the general decline in diphtheria morbidity.

Could Diptheria Return?

The report of a serious case of diphtheria in a Finnish man, contracted during a trip to Russia, has resuscitated interest in the need for booster vaccinations (22). This particular patient entered hospital during Easter 1993, developed neurological symptoms (paraesthesia of right mandibular area and loss of power in all four extremities) and signs of myocardial toxicity. He was still in hospital at the time of the publication of the case (July 1993). The absence of the toxinogenic strains in countries where inoculation was widespread means that one does not acquire booster protection by natural infection. It may thus be necessary to reinforce protection, particularly for those travelling to countries endemic for diphtheria. The non-toxic, antigenic cross reacting materials (CRM), obtained after random mutagenesis of the TOX gene, may be developed as suitable alternatives to the toxoid vaccines (23), which may cause untoward reactions in adults.

The occasional case of diphtheria that occurs intermittently in Europe, serious as each is, serves as a reminder of how far we have progressed from the dire situation in the diphtheria wards one hundred years ago.

An earlier version of this chapter was published as: Diphtheria – understanding, treatment and prevention. RDS News January 1994 8-12.

References

1) Whitelegge BA, Newman G (1893) *Hygiene and Public Health*. 2nd ed, London: Cassell.

2) Roux E, Yersin A (1888) Contribution à l'étude de la diphthérie. *Ann l'Inst Pasteur* 2 629-61.

3) Behring von E, Kitasato S (1890) Ueber das Zustandekommen der Diphtherie-Immunität und der Tetanus-Immunität bei Thieren. *Deutsch Med Wochensch* **16** 1113-14.

4) Zinsser H (1931) *Textbook of Bacteriology*. 6th ed, New York: Appleton.

5) Roux ME, Martin ML & Chaillou MA (1894) Trois cents cas de diphtérie traités par le sérum antidiphtérique. *Ann l'Inst Pasteur* **8** 640-61.

6) Paget S (1906) *Experiments on Animals*, 2nd ed, London: Nisbet.

7) Beddow Bayly M (1934) *The Schick Inoculation for Immunisation against Diphtheria*. BUAV and the National Anti-Vaccination League.

8) Rogers L (1937) *The Truth About Vivisection*. London: Churchill.

9) (1899) Report of the Special Committee on Diphtheria Antitoxin. *Trans Clin Soc* **31** 1-50.

10) Cobbett L (1933) The decline in the death rate of diphtheria compared with that of scarlet fever. *BMJ* ii 139-40.

11) Behring von E (1913) Ueber ein neues Diphtherieschutzmittel. *Deutsch Med Wochenschr* **39** 873-76.

12) Glenny AT & Hopkins BE (1923) Diphtheria toxoid as an immunising agent. *Br J Exp Pathol* **4** 283-288. http://www.ncbi.nlm.nih.gov/pmc/articles/PMC2047731/

13) Ramon G (1924) Sur la toxine et sur l'anatoxine diphthiriques. *Ann l'Inst Pasteur* **38** 1-10.

14) (1953) Diphtheria and Pertussis Vaccination WHO Technical Report Series No 61. http://whqlibdoc.who.int/trs/WHO_TRS_61.pdf

15) Harries EH (1939) Control of the common fevers: diphtheria. *The Lancet* i 45-48.

16) (1932) Report of Society of Medical Officers of Health. *The Medical Officer* **48** 188.

17) Burn M & Fellowes V (1934) Diphtheria immunisation: a review of eight years work in Birmingham. *The Lancet* ii 1181-85.

18) Clayton Smith A (1932) Letter to *Yorkshire Observer*, May 17.

19) Clayton Smith A (1932) Letter to *Yorkshire Observer*, May 24.

20) Greenwood Wilson J (MOH, Dewsbury) (1932) Letter to *Yorkshire Observer*, May 21.

21) WHO (1951) Epidemiology and Vital Statistics Report. **4** 92-111.

22) Lumio J, Jahkola M, Vuento R, Haikala O & Eskola J (1993) Diphtheria after visit to Russia. *The Lancet* **342** 53-54.

23) Cryz SJ (1991) *Vaccines and Immunotherapy*. New York: Pergamon.

II. DEVELOPMENT OF LIFE-SAVING PROCEDURES

8. Development of Dialysis to Treat Loss of Kidney Function

The kidney regulates the water, acid/alkali and ion balance of the body, and removes toxic products of metabolism and ingested poisons. It is thus not surprising that when the kidney fails to function properly the consequences are dire. Urine production falls and toxins build up in the plasma ultimately producing coma. Cardiac arrhythmias may be induced through build-up of potassium ions in the plasma. Death results if the condition is severe and untreated.

Acute renal failure is a sudden decline in renal function as a result of poisoning or reduced cardiac output (due to severe haemorrhage, shock, septicaemia, myocardial infarction etc.). Chronic renal failure (CRF), due to pyelonephritis, glomerulonephritis, hypertension or diabetes, is characterised by a more gradual loss of function. The chronic disease can be controlled to some extent by a low sodium, low protein diet. But both for acute renal failure, and for the 5,000 patients per year in the UK that develop *chronic* renal failure, the life-saving technique of dialysis is essential.

Haemodialysis

The crucial discovery in the development of dialysis techniques was that of Thomas Graham, who in 1854 showed that colloids and crystalloids could be separated in aqueous solution. Graham demonstrated the movement of urea and sodium chloride, but not colloids, through a semipermeable membrane (treated parchment, 1). Over the next 50 years, collodion became the most popular material for the formation of a semipermeable membrane and Richardson must receive credit for being the first to suggest that

http://dx.doi.org/10.11647/OBP.0055.08

animal blood could be "dialysed" by passing it through a colloidal tube surrounded by saline (2).

The first practical demonstration of the continuous dialysis of blood outside the body (i.e. in an "extracorporeal circuit") was performed by Abel and his co-workers (3). They took blood from arteries of chloretone-anaesthetised dogs and rabbits and passed it through a series of celloidin tubes immersed in saline (celloidin was a brand of collodion). The blood was then returned to the animal *via* a cannulated vein. The animals made complete recoveries after being subjected to this "vividiffusion" for 2-3 hours.

Abel did not actually develop the apparatus as a prototype machine for treating renal failure. His main interest was the measurement of the plasma concentration of physiologically active substances such as hormones. Detection of these in the plasma was difficult since they were often lost during precipitation of the plasma proteins, to which they could adhere. Abel thus hoped that this form of dialysis would extract active substances as fast as they entered the blood, without at the same time removing proteins and cells. Nevertheless Abel stated in his paper that the machine might act as an "artificial kidney" which might be used to tide over a dangerous crisis in one of the:

> numerous toxic states in which the eliminating organs, more especially the kidneys, are incapable of removing from the body at an adequate rate, either the autochthonous or the foreign substances whose presence in excessive amount is detrimental to life processes.

Abel prevented coagulation in the extracorporeal circulation by the use of the anticoagulant extracted from leeches, hirudin (Hirudin, at $27.50 per gram, appears to have been the 1913 equivalent of some of the contemporary, expensive recombinant-produced proteins. Abel therefore extracted hirudin for himself from leeches bought from cupping barbers at the rate of $6 per hundred).

Anticoagulants and Cellophane

It was difficult to extract large quantities of hirudin for use in haemodialysis, and the early preparations were very impure and caused severe cardiovascular-respiratory side effects and allergic reactions. This meant that such preparations could only be used for animal studies. The absence of a suitable anticoagulant to prevent blood clotting in the extracorporeal circuits prevented the clinical use of haemodialysis. The despair and frustration experienced by military physicians during World War I, observing the inevitable death of troops from renal failure following severe traumatic damage, ensured the continued experimental investigation of the technique. More efficient dialysis membranes were prepared, and the design of dialysis machines was modified so that a smaller volume of blood was required to fill the extra corporeal circuit. A significant event was the commercial manufacture of long lengths of cellophane tubing. Although prepared originally as sausage casings, their potential as dialysis membranes in artificial kidney machines was soon recognised.

The discovery of the anticoagulant that occurred naturally in mammals, heparin, was a turning point in the clinical use of dialysis. Heparin was isolated from dog liver by McLean in 1916, when he was actually trying to prepare clotting factors (4). Haas produced a batch of heparin in 1925 and showed that it performed well during dialysis in his animal studies (5). But as with hirudin, the early extracts of heparin were very impure and could not be used in patients. However, the relative abundance of heparin, large amounts of which could be extracted from beef liver and lung, meant that biochemists were free to experiment with purification techniques. In 1937 Murray(6), using purified extracts (250 units/mg) produced by Charles and Scott, showed that injection of heparin into dogs, rabbits, guinea pigs and mice rendered their blood incoagulable for long periods with no apparent ill effects. A sample of double the purity (500 units/mg) was then administered to patients with "no deleterious effects" (6).

Heparin was thus used as the anticoagulant in the first successful treatment of a patient in acute renal failure by the Dutchman Willem Kolff in 1945.[1] Although she was completely comatose when the treatment was initiated, the use of the artificial kidney designed by Kolff brought her out of the coma. Renal function improved and she survived. The life-saving potential of dialysis was realised (5).

Heparin must still be prepared from animal sources, *viz* the lungs of oxen or the intestinal mucosa of oxen, sheep or pigs. Like many substances

---

1 "One of my first patients was a young man suffering from chronic nephritis and slowly dying of renal failure. He was hypertensive, had headaches, became blind, and was vomiting every day. His old mother was the wife of a poor farmer, her back bent by hard work, dressed in her traditional Sunday black dress, but with a very pretty white lace cap. I had to tell her that her only son was going to die, and I felt very helpless." Dr Willem Kolff, the first person to treat a patient with an artificial kidney. Written in a letter to Dr F. D. Moore, quoted in F. D. Moore, *Give and Take: The Development of Tissue Transplantation*. Philadelphia: Saunders.

extracted from animal tissue, the safety of each batch must be ensured by testing samples on an anaesthetised animal to ensure the absence of substances that may lower blood pressure (7).

Alternative Anticoagulants

Even in the presence of heparin, blood platelets can deposit on the dialysis membranes and thus cause a thrombocytopenia (fall in platelet levels) in the patient. Some low molecular weight fragments of heparin are anticoagulant and are said to produce less of a fall in platelet levels. Such compounds may be of use in dialysis in patients with a high bleeding risk.

Epoprostenol (prostacyclin) is an endogenous prostanoid made by the innermost cells of the blood vessels. Its ability to prevent platelet aggregation *in vivo* was demonstrated in a number of species (8). Epoprostenol was shown to be capable of replacing heparin in dialysis in anaesthetised dogs (9). Subsequent tests in dialysis patients showed that with small amounts of epoprostenol, the dose of heparin could be reduced to avoid problems in high-bleeding-risk patients. Epoprostenol thus has a guaranteed place in the management of dialysis where haemorrhage may be a problem.

Rather belatedly, highly purified samples of the first anticoagulant, hirudin, have now become available. Studies in dogs, rabbits and rats showed hirudin to be well-tolerated with low toxicity. The cardiovascular-respiratory effects seen in dogs with the partially purified hirudin were not seen with the highly purified preparations (10). Subsequent tests of the purified hirudin samples in healthy volunteers showed that they were also innocuous to humans (11). (It is of interest that the pharmacokinetic data, i.e. plasma half-life and urinary excretion of unchanged hirudin, were virtually the same in both animal and human studies).

Since hirudin can now be produced in recombinant form, it is possible that it may, after 100 years, find a use in dialysis.

Peritoneal Dialysis

Wegner, in 1877, was the first to conduct experiments into the effect of placing solutions of various concentrations into the peritoneal space (12). He noted that if a particular volume of a concentrated sugar solution was injected into the peritoneum of rabbits, a larger volume could be subsequently withdrawn.

Changes in volume and osmotic pressure of fluids placed in the peritoneal space were further studied by Starling and his co-workers between 1894 and 1895. In the same species they noted that on injection of hypotonic solutions their volume in the peritoneum decreased within hours, but when an isotonic solution was used, the volume remained the same for 2-3 hours (actually the fluid began to be absorbed after this time). The inevitable conclusion was that the serous surfaces of the peritoneum behaved as an inert membrane, the volume of fluid within the peritoneal cavity being dependent on the osmotic pressure on either side of the membrane (13).

It was natural to assume that small molecules might cross the peritoneal membranes, the rate of passage depending on the relative concentrations in the blood or the peritoneal fluid. From the 1920s to 1930s, experiments on rabbits, dogs and monkeys showed that the peritoneal membranes were permeable to most low molecular weight substances (including urea) and even some proteins (13). Warming the solutions placed in the peritoneum, and increasing the movement of the gut were found to accelerate the diffusion of substances out of the blood into the fluid in the peritoneum.

The conclusion derived from these animal experiments was that if fluid was placed in the space surrounding the highly vascular intestines, the membranes between the blood and the injected solution acted in the same way as the artificial membrane in vividiffusion. That is, they allowed low molecular weight substances to diffuse across to an area of low concentration.

Peritoneal Dialysis in Uraemic Animals

It was a natural assumption that it would be possible to remove waste products from the blood into suitable solutions injected into the peritoneum. Experiments were therefore performed on uraemic animals. Solutions were either placed in the peritoneum, left for a sufficient time and then replaced with a fresh solution, or a continuous method was used. In this case the solution was caused to flow into the peritoneum through one catheter and allowed to drain out through a second.

Ganter in 1923 performed peritoneal dialysis on guinea pigs and rabbits with anuria (and hence uraemia) induced by ligation of the ureters. Constant, intraperitoneal injection of 50 ml samples of a physiological salt solution produced a marked clinical improvement. The animals became less lethargic and began walking around in search of food (14).

Later investigations were virtually restricted to tests on bilaterally nephrectomised dogs. Such experiments clearly demonstrated that peritoneal dialysis could prolong the life of uraemic dogs from a control level of 3-5 days, to 13 (15), 70 (16) and even 111 days (17). Through such experiments the optimal formulations of the dialysis solutions were derived and possible complications of the procedure exposed. One such was peritonitis, and as a consequence antibiotics were added to dialysis fluids used for patients from 1957 onwards.

These early animal experiments laid the basis for the use of peritoneal dialysis for the removal of toxins from the blood of patients. The use of peritoneal dialysis gradually intensified from 1945 onwards with constant refinements being added to the technique. Continuous ambulatory peritoneal dialysis (CAPD), in which waste products and water are continuously removed whilst patients carry on with their normal activities, became freely available in the UK in 1980.

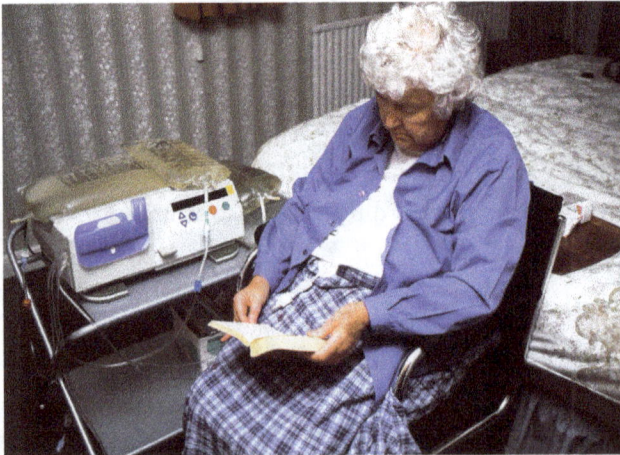

Fig. 8.1 In the 1960s, the NHS only supplied dialysis for acute kidney failure; patients with chronic kidney failure had to pay about £7,000 for machines and technical support. However, today kidney dialysis machines like these are widely available. © Science Photo Library, all rights reserved.

Anaemia During Dialysis: Erythropoietin

Another problem associated with renal failure is anaemia. This is not secondary to the dialysis, but to the fact that the diseased kidney is not able to produce a factor that normally promotes the maturation of red blood cells, erythropoietin (EPO). Our knowledge of the importance of EPO and other agents in the prevention of anaemia stems originally from studies of the circulating haemopoietic factors that appear in the blood of anaemic rabbits (18). The kidney was shown to be the main site of formation of EPO after experiments in rats and rabbits which demonstrated a sharp fall in plasma EPO activity after nephrectomy, but no change after removal of other organs (19). Defective production of EPO in patients in chronic renal failure can render some patients dependent on regular blood transfusions. EPO can now be prepared by recombinant methods and it is highly effective for the treatment of the anaemia of chronic renal failure, removing the requirement for transfusion within weeks.

Dialysis without question saves the lives of patients with acute and chronic renal failure. The basic animal research, performed around the turn of the century, exposed the possibility of removal of toxic metabolites from the blood by diffusion across semipermeable membranes. Without those experiments, the 100 patients per million population per annum (20) that develop CRF would have no future. However, while dialysis is life-saving, the treatment for CRF with the best prognosis is a kidney transplant (21). Transplantation is also the most cost effective treatment (20).

An earlier version of this chapter was published as: Development of dialysis to treat loss of kidney function. *RDS News* January 1995 8-11.

References

1) Graham T (1854) Osmotic force. *Philo Trans Roy Soc. London* **144** 177-228.

2) Richardson B (1889) Practical studies in animal dialysis. *Asclepiad* **6** 331-32.

3) Abel J, Rowntree L, Turner B (1914) Plasma removal with return of corpuscles (Plasmaphaeresis). *J Pharmacol Exp Ther* **5** 275-316.

4) Beck E. (1984) The treatment of thrombosis, in *Discoveries in Pharmacology*, vol. 2, eds Parnham M & Bruinvels J. Amsterdam: Elsevier.

5) McBride P (1980) The Development of hemodialysis and peritoneal dialysis, in *Clinical Dialysis*, eds Nissenson A, Fine R & Gentile D. Englewood Cliffs: Prentice-Hall.

6) Murray D, Jaques M, Perrett T & Best C (1937) Heparin and thrombosis of veins following surgery. *Surgery* **2** 163-87.

7) Department of Health *The British Pharmacopoeia*. London: Stationery Office Books 1993.

8) Gryglewski R, Botting R & Vane J (1988) Mediators produced by the endothelial cell. *Hypertens* **12** 530-548

9) Woods H, Ash G, Weston M, Bunting S, Moncada S & Vane J (1978) Prostacyclin can replace heparin in haemodialysis in dogs. *The Lancet* **2** 1075-77.

10) Markwardt F, Hauptmann J, Nowak G, Klessen C & Walsmann P (1982) Pharmacological studies on the antithrombotic action of Hirudin in experimental animals. *Thromb Haemostas* **47** 226-29.

11) Markwardt F, Nowak G, Stuerzebecher J Griessbach U, Walsmann P & Vogel G (1984) Pharmacokinetics and anticoagulant effect of hirudin in man. *Thromb Haemostas* **52** 160-63.

12) Wegner G (1877) Chirurgische Bemerkungen über die Peritonealhöhle, mit besonderer Berücksichtigung der Ovariotomie. *Arch f klin Chir* **20** 51-55.

13) Boen S (1964) *Peritoneal Dialysis in Clinical Medicine*. Springfield: Charles Thomas.

14) Ganter G (1923) Ueber die Beseitigung giftiger Stoffe aus dem Blute durch Dialyse. *Muench Med Wochschr* **70** 1478.

15) Bliss S, Kastler A, Nadler S (1931) Peritoneal lavage. Effective elimination of nitrogenous wastes in the absence of kidney function. *Proc Soc Exp Biol and Med* **29** 1078-79.

16) Grollman A, Turner L & Mclean J (1951) Intermittent peritoneal lavage in nephrectomised dogs and its application to the human being. *Arch Int Med* **87** 379.

17) Houck C, More A, ElksonW & Gilmer R (1954) Intestinal intussusception in chronic nephrectomised dogs maintained by peritoneal dialysis. *Science* June **11** 845.

18) Carnot P & Deflandre O (1906) Sur l'activite hemopoietique du serum. *Compt rend Acad d Sc Par* **143** 384-86.

19) Jacobson L, Goldwasser E, Fried W & Plzak L (1957) Role of the kidney in erythropoiesis. *Nature* **179** 633-34.

20) West R (1991) *Organ Transplantation*. London: Office of Health Economics.

21) Minerva (1993) *Br Med J* **307** 880.

9. The Contribution of Animal Experiments to Kidney Transplantation

Haemodialysis is life-saving and curative in acute renal failure. By reversing the build-up of metabolic products normally excreted by a functioning kidney, dialysis enables the temporarily affected kidneys to heal and resume normal function. In chronic renal failure however, the burden of regular dialysis is necessary unless a healthy kidney from a donor can be grafted.

Chronic Renal Failure

Chronic renal failure (CRF) due to glomerulonephritis, pyelonephritis or polycystic kidney disease is quite common, particularly in young adults. Depending on the composition of the population, between 50 and 100 persons per million will develop chronic renal failure each year (1).

In the absence of treatment, the deterioration in kidney function results in anaemia and weakness. Since water cannot be excreted, fluid accumulates in the tissues and consequent lung oedema causes breathing difficulties and strain on the heart, an organ probably already compromised by high blood pressure, which is a common feature of kidney failure. The build-up of waste products results in inflammation of various tissues leading to pericarditis, colitis, diarrhoea, gastritis and persistent vomiting. Peripheral neuritis can result in paralysis (2).

Experiments in Transplantation

The miserable clinical picture of the patient, often young, sinking inexorably into coma, and from coma to death was a potent stimulus to research. The

http://dx.doi.org/10.11647/OBP.0055.09

possibility of treating CRF by grafting a healthy kidney was a natural experiment to attempt. However, the transplantation of a large organ such as the kidney, which receives its blood supply *via* a single, large artery, requires the connection (or anastomosis) of the renal artery and vein of the donor kidney with a suitable artery and vein in the patient. This was no simple task since the arterial anastomosis had to be secure enough to withstand systolic blood pressure.

This formidable problem was resolved by the French surgeon Alexis Carrel (Fig. 9.1), who in 1902 described a method for suturing together the cut ends of blood vessels (3).

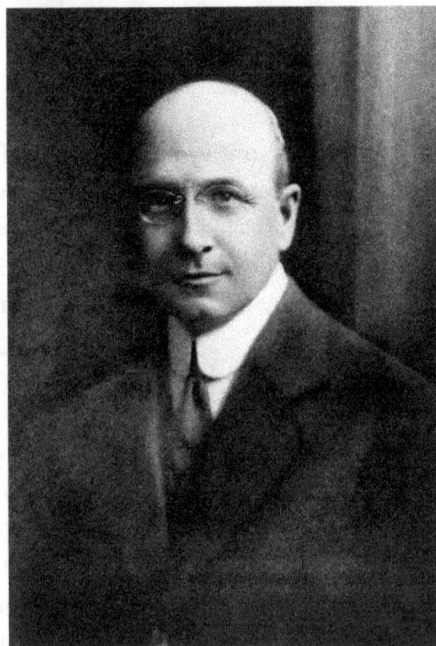

Fig. 9.1 Alexis Carrel, 1912 Nobel Laureate in Physiology or Medicine. Wellcome Library, London, CC BY.

Carrel initially fixed three sutures equidistant around the end of each vessel and applied tension, thus forming a triangle. Corresponding sides of the triangulated vessels were then sewn together using extremely fine needles and the thinnest linen thread as used by the lace makers of Valenciennes (Fig. 9. 2). Carrel performed many anastomoses, of various types, in cats and dogs. These healed and functioned well for many months (4). It is noteworthy that

Carrel emphasised the importance of protecting the endothelial cell layer during the procedure. A fact he found by experiment, but obvious today in view of the many important factors known to be synthesised and released by these cells.

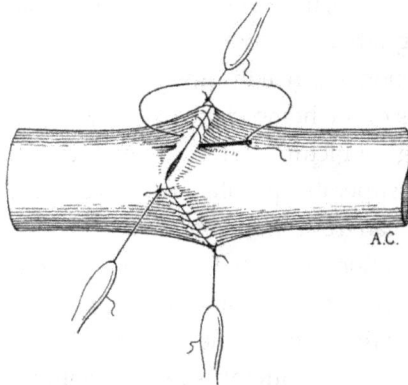

Fig. 9.2 Carrel's vascular anastamosis. From A. Carrel (1902), 'La Technique operatoire des anastomoses vasculaire et la transplantation des visceres', *Medecine de Lyon*, 98, 859.

Carrel used his suturing technique to experiment with kidney transplantation in dog and cat. His anastomoses enabled a kidney, removed and transplanted to a different site in the same animal (an autograft), to function adequately provided that the organ was not deprived of a blood supply for too long. However, a kidney grafted from another animal of the same species (a homograft or allograft) functioned for only a few days. After that it would become oedematous and cease to work. After many experiments, Carrel became convinced that it was not the surgery that caused the problem, since autografts always functioned reasonably well. He concluded that the changes that occurred in the kidney transplanted from a different animal of the same species were due to "biological factors" from the host. Thus the phenomenon of rejection was exposed (5).

Rejection

Carrel was the first scientist in America to be awarded the Nobel Prize. This was in 1912 for work on "vasculature suture and transplantation of organs." He returned to France at the outbreak of World War I. Although he went back to the USA in 1919, he did not return to the problem of kidney transplantation, but worked on the *in vitro* cultivation of organs and tissues.

The inevitability of the rejection of homografted kidneys was confirmed in 1923 by Williamson, a surgeon working at the Mayo Clinic Foundation. Williamson's experiments in dogs were similar to those of Carrel. They were slightly more sophisticated, however, in that he analysed the urine produced by the kidney homografts and autografts, and noted that there was very little difference until rejection began in the homograft. Williamson also examined microscopic sections of the homografted kidneys and was thus the first to describe the histological picture of the kidney during rejection (6).

The seemingly insuperable problem of the refusal by a host to tolerate the presence of an organ from another animal from the same species caused a hiatus in transplantation research. It was not for another 20 years that the dreary clinical picture, and the frustration of the physician attempting to treat CRF, again stimulated research into the possibility of kidney transplantation.

There were some sporadic attempts to transplant kidneys into seriously ill patients. The thigh was usually chosen as the transplant site. This was anatomically inconvenient, but the ease of access meant that the kidney could be easily examined and removed without major surgery. As might have been predicted, long-term survival was not attained.[1]

Perfection of the Surgery

Although, in experimental animal studies, autografted kidneys worked adequately, they did not function in a completely normal way. This was probably due to the absence of the nerve supply, lymphatic drainage and various other factors. The surgeon Joseph Murray joined the Brigham Hospital in Boston in 1951, and initially worked in the laboratory to determine the optimum surgical technique for kidney transplantation. Murray demonstrated in dog that the best place for the graft was in the abdomen, behind the peritoneal membrane and connected to the blood vessels of the pelvis. The ureter could then be

---

1   One surprising example of a homotransplanted kidney surviving for 175 days without any immunosuppressive therapy is described by Moore (The case of "Dr. W" in Ref. 7). The patient ultimately died as a result of severe hypertension, the kidney showing no classical sign of rejection. There is no explanation for this random success. It was an early example of the occasional apparent acceptance of a graft that occurs in both animal and human experiments, perhaps due to a chance close tissue matching.

sutured to the bladder, instead of to the skin, as in the early transplants (the latter technique frequently resulted in infection). By 1954 Murray had several dogs living for over 2 years on a life-sustaining renal autograft (7).

Armed with a perfected technique, and impressed with the knowledge that a kidney allograft in a dog with both kidneys removed would excrete urine and support life until rejection, the surgeons at the Brigham began in earnest to attempt transplantation in patients with CRF. Without any attempt to tackle the problem of rejection these were obviously not successful. Nevertheless important lessons were learned. As in the animal studies, the transplanted kidney could restore the uraemic patient to normal and Murray's placement of the kidney in the abdomen, and the anastomosis with pelvic vessels perfected in dog, worked well in patients. The necessity of sometimes removing the diseased kidneys to prevent hypertension was established, and the pathological changes occurring in the kidney during rejection were observed and shown to be similar to those in the animal studies.

The Mechanism of Rejection: An Immunological Phenomenon

Clues to the mechanism of the rejection of homografted tissue had actually appeared in the literature long before surgeons were seriously considering kidney grafting for CRF.

In 1916 Little and Tyzzer (8) had shown that tumours that arose spontaneously in one strain of mice could be transplanted to other individual mice within that strain, but not to mice of a different strain, who would reject them. Gorer, in 1937 (9), used similar experiments to demonstrate that the rejection of a tumour inherent to one mouse strain by mice of another strain was due to tissue antigen(s) (designated by Gorer as antigen II). This could raise tumour-destructive antibodies that would also agglutinate red cells of the tumour strain of mice.

The definitive analysis of the immunological nature of graft rejection was provided by Medawar (Fig. 9.3) and his co-workers. The need to treat severe burns incurred by both service personnel and civilians during World War II prompted the British government to sponsor a study of skin grafting. Medawar, in conjunction with a plastic surgeon, studied the use of skin autografts and homografts for burns. Initially both grafts seemed to take, but after a few days the allograft began to darken and die. Further allografts from the same donor were rejected even more rapidly. This became known as the "second set phenomenon" and was the observation that caused Medawar to conclude that the rejection of allografts was brought about by active immunisation (10).

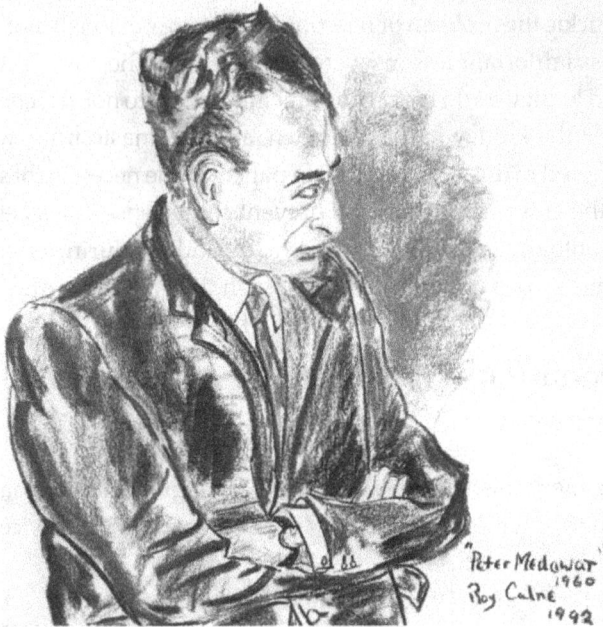

Fig. 9.3 Sir Peter Medawar, painting by Sir Roy Calne.

On his return to Oxford University after the war Medawar continued with his classic experiments which ultimately resulted in his Nobel Prize of 1960. Medawar and his colleagues set up an animal model to examine the mechanism of rejection of skin grafts under tightly controlled conditions. He grafted skin between rabbits and established the control data of average times to rejection. Repeated grafts from the same donors were rejected much more quickly, whereas grafts from a *second* donor lasted as long as the initial grafts. Medawar thus had illustrated clearly the specificity of graft rejection. He also made careful histological examinations of the grafts and described their invasion by the white blood cells. This established beyond doubt the immunological nature of the rejection reaction (7).

Prevention of Rejection: An Impossible Goal?

During the 1930s the concept of genetic individuality had emerged. Loeb, in his book *The Biological Basis of Individuality*, stated that any transplant between individuals would inevitably fail, since there were differences in the genetic make-up of everyone. Twenty years later, Loeb was invited to an international conference on transplantation. He declined, since he considered that "the subject matter of the conference was useless to pursue and a waste of time because the goal was impossible"(11). Unfortunately such emphatic assertions tend to be recorded in perpetuity. Since today there are patients with kidney transplants of more than 20 years standing, this provides a lesson for those tempted to make definitive statements based on intuition rather than evidence.

Experimental work during the 1950s increased our knowledge of immune mechanisms and strengthened the view that the rejection reaction might be capable of modification, so that transplants could succeed.

The fact that two genetic types could coexist in the same organism, without rejection of either, emerged from studies in cattle twins. Twinning is rare in cattle, and identical twinning is virtually unknown. In a study of cattle twins, Owen (12) noted that each twin carried blood cells of two different types. The fact that each was tolerated was presumed to be the result of an admixture of bloods between the twins *in utero* (Lillie, in 1916, had shown that in bovine twins there was often a union of the circulatory systems between the two placentae) (13).

The inevitable conclusion of these observations was that exposure to genetically dissimilar cells during fetal life rendered cells of that type *tolerable* in later life.

Other animal experiments consolidated this conclusion. Cannon and Longmire (14) transplanted skin between newly hatched (one-day-old) chicks of different breeds, producing adult red hens with patches of skin growing white feathers (in later experiments they also reversed the position of the skin, so that the white feathers were projecting in a different direction to the rest of the plumage). Delaying the skin graft for three days reduced the success rate to 1%, at 14 days all grafts were rejected.

Medawar also experimented with younger and younger animals, and in 1953 published a significant paper describing what he termed as "actively acquired tolerance" (as opposed to actively acquired immunity) (15). Medawar and his co-workers anaesthetised a mouse (CBA strain), pregnant and near to term. By a careful incision they exposed the abdominal body wall. The fetuses were sequentially brought into view by gentle manipulation of the abdomen and injected with a suspension of cells from adult mice of a different strain (A-line). Eight weeks after birth, each member of the CBA litter received a skin graft from an A-line mouse. The grafts took satisfactorily and resulted in the much-photographed mice carrying patches of fur of an entirely different colour. Medawar had thus shown that exposure of mice *in utero* to tissue of a genetically different strain produced a tolerance to that tissue.

Although "actively acquired tolerance," as experimentally accomplished by Medawar, had no immediate application to the problem of rejection of kidney grafts, this work demonstrated that the immunological barrier was not insuperable. This was immensely encouraging for the surgeons endeavouring to achieve long-term survival of transplanted kidneys. (One such surgeon recorded his debt to Medawar in his account of the history of organ transplantation (16)).

The Identical Twins: A Vindication of the Surgery

It was evident that rejection of grafts would be unlikely if the organ or tissue came from an identical twin, since such monozygotic twins were also genetically identical. As everyone possesses a pair of kidneys, the surgeons at the Brigham Hospital had long considered that the donation of one kidney from a healthy twin might well be life-saving for the other suffering from CRF. The opportunity to put this to the test arose in 1953, when "Mr R H" was admitted to the Boston Public Health Service Hospital with chronic nephritis. His illness was severe and the outlook poor. Upon learning that the patient had a twin brother, his physician contacted the Brigham Hospital to suggest that this might be a case for a successful transplantation. Having ascertained that the tissue of the twins was interchangeable (by cross grafting patches of skin), and after establishing that the potential donor had a healthy urinary system, the question as to whether the transplant should be attempted was seriously addressed by the scientific and surgical team at the Brigham.

At a meeting on 20 December 1954 it was decided to proceed with the operation and, in view of Doctor Murray's experience with dogs, to place the donated kidney in the abdomen with the ureter anastomosed directly to the bladder (7).

The operation was performed on December 23, 1954. The transplanted kidney began to produce "crystal clear normal urine" before the surgeons even had time to sew the severed ureter to the bladder. The patient recovered rapidly after the operation. His heart, which had been enlarged, returned to normal size, fluid cleared from his lungs and he was returned to health. Mr RH married the nurse who had tended him in hospital and raised a family.

To attempt this first identical twin transplant was a brave action by the medical team at the Brigham. It showed unequivocally that in man, as in dog, this operation was feasible and that the transplanted organ performed normally. Attention then turned to the apparently insuperable problem of maintaining grafts from genetically different donors.

Whole Body Irradiation

Intense radiation was known to be particularly toxic to the mediators of rejection, the white blood cells. In view of the implacability of the problem it was not surprising that even this drastic procedure was examined as a means of prolonging survival of grafted kidneys. High levels of x-radiation were shown to prolong the life of skin homografts in rabbits, but at the cost of shortening the life of the host, since damage to the bone marrow rendered the animals susceptible to infection (17). Researchers tried to combat this problem by subsequent administration of homologous and heterologous bone marrow cells. The survival time of mice exposed to lethal x-radiation was increased by such treatment. Subsequently, skin grafts between rabbits showed extended survival after x-radiation and injection of hybrid bone marrow prior to grafting (18).

A successful renal graft was achieved in an irradiated dog at the Mary Imogene Bassett Hospital in Cooperstown. The animal was infused with bone marrow from the donor animal. Unfortunately the lack of an effective immune system resulted in the death of the animal from pneumonia after 49 days. However the grafted kidney functioned excellently for this period, with no sign of rejection (19).

The results of these animal experiments did not really augur well for the value of x-radiation in patients in need of a kidney graft. However, dire situations produce drastic action. X-radiation followed by administration of bone marrow from numerous relatives was used to prevent rejection of a kidney graft in a woman who had her only kidney removed to stem a life-threatening haemorrhage. After some while her platelet levels dropped and, perhaps predictably, she died of haemorrhage 32 days after the irradiation. Of great significance however, at the post mortem the kidney showed no sign of rejection (7).

Despite one apparent success, where the kidney was donated from a fraternal twin, and hence only a low level of radiation was used, the toxic effects of the radiation in patients, as in the animals, rendered this technique too dangerous. Nevertheless, the continued functioning of the transplanted kidneys did encourage the surgeons to believe that prevention of rejection was achievable (7).

Success with the First Immunosuppressants

A paper of great significance in transplant research is that of Robert Schwartz and William Dameshek of Tufts University Medical School. These workers showed, in 1959, that the anticancer drug 6-mercaptopurine (6-MP) given to rabbits, prevented the formation of antibodies following the injection of human serum albumin (20). In other words, 6-MP was capable of suppressing an immune response. Within one year Schwartz and Dameshek had extended this work to show that 6-MP could triple the survival time of skin homografts in rabbits (21).

The British surgeon, Roy Calne demonstrated the value of 6-MP in delaying the rejection of kidney allografts in dogs. In his first series of experiments, although 6 mg of 6-MP per day prevented rejection, the animals died within 10-14 days. In a second series, the animals were bilaterally nephrectomised (and thus had to depend solely on the graft) and were given 5 mg of 6-MP initially. This was reduced to 2.5 mg after 2 days. Incredibly, two dogs survived for 21 and 47 days respectively. Without 6-MP dogs so treated would survive only 4 to 8 days, and ultimately die of kidney failure. Both of the test dogs died of pneumonia. The kidneys, however, showed no sign of rejection and were secreting concentrated urine to the end (22).

Calne at this time joined the active team at the Brigham Hospital for a sabbatical, where a collaboration was formed with the synthetic chemists at the Burroughs Wellcome Research laboratories in Tuckahoe, New York. These researchers, under the leadership of Dr George Hitchings, synthesised new analogues of 6-MP and produced azathioprine, orally active and less toxic than 6-MP. With azathioprine it was possible to keep bilaterally nephrectomised dogs alive for up to 12 months (Fig. 9.4), dependent only on their grafted kidney (7). This experimental work led to the use of immunosuppressant drugs in patients with kidney grafts. From 1963 onward one-year survival of related donor transplants reached 80%.

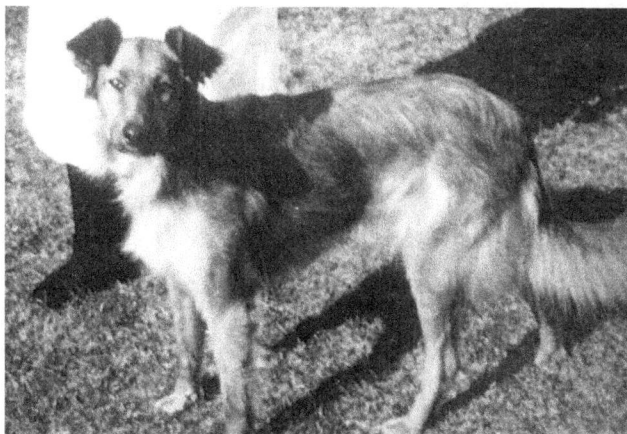

Fig. 9.4 The first long-surviving dog, Lollypop, treated with the immunosuppressant azathioprine following a kidney graft. All rights reserved.

Corticosteroids, such as cortisone and the newer synthetic analogues, soon began to be used in conjunction with azathioprine. Corticosteroids were known to inhibit antigen-antibody reactions and were subsequently shown to produce a threefold increase in the survival time of dog kidney homografts (23).

In the late 1970s cyclosporin was extracted from the fungus *Tolypocladium inflatum*, and purified as a potential antifungal agent. It was however, shown to be rather better as a potent immunosuppressant in animal tests. It suppressed the appearance of plaque-forming cells in the spleens of mice immunised with sheep red blood cells, and doubled the survival time of skin allografts in mice. Cyclosporin has become established as a front-line immunosuppressant drug.

Antilymphocyte Serum

Since the lymphocyte is the cell primarily responsible for rejection, it is not surprising that antilymphocyte serum (ALS) has been developed as a potential antirejection agent. Metchnikoff in 1899 was the first to prepare ALS by injecting guinea pigs with extracts of rat or rabbit lymph nodes (25). The sera produced caused agglutination of rat or rabbit white cells. Woodruff clearly demonstrated the benefit of ALS in transplantation by showing it produced a ten-fold increase in survival time of skin homografts between albino and hooded rats (26). Despite problems of standardisation, ALS raised in horses is used in acute rejection crises. Poor tolerance to horse proteins, manifested by some patients, necessitates the occasional use of ALS raised in rabbits.

Tissue Typing

The genetic basis of rejection had been exposed by the mouse tumour transplant experiments of Little and Tyzzer (*vide supra*). The use of inbred strains of mice differing at only a single genetic locus from the original strain (congenic strains) enabled Gorer and Snell to establish the genetic locus (the "H" locus) for transplantation antigens. This work on the murine counterpart of human leucocyte antigens (HLA) hastened the understanding of transplantation antigens and emphasised the need for adequate tissue typing to ensure the best chance of long-term survival of kidney grafts (27)

The Future

Despite the emphatic progress made in organ transplantation, there is still need for improvement in antirejection therapy. Tacrolimus (FK 506) was introduced in 1989 but seems to share the same toxic effects as cyclosporin. Using transplant models in rodents, dogs and monkeys various groups of researchers have produced many candidate antirejection drugs (28). It is estimated that at the moment there are 10 novel non-peptide drugs and 15 monoclonal antibodies in various stages of clinical and preclinical testing (28). From this research will no doubt come further, step-by-step improvements in immunosuppressive therapy.

The continual improvements in methods to prevent rejection have resulted in an increase in patients on the waiting list for a transplant. The shortage of donors has thus become the major problem, exacerbated by the fall in donors resulting from improved road safety measures.

This problem would be eased if kidneys from another species (xenotransplants) could be used. A colony of transgenic pigs has now been produced which possess human genes intended to protect the transplant against the acute, complement driven, rejection process that normally occurs with xenotransplants. The first transplant from a pig to a human will no doubt be attempted within the next decade.

About 2,000 patients per year receive a kidney transplant in the UK (Figs. 9.5 and 9.6). Over two-thirds of these can expect their grafts to survive for at least a decade (1). In his admirable history of tissue transplantation, Francis Moore (then Professor of Surgery at Harvard) stated that none of the advances in kidney transplantation could have occurred without the extensive research in animals (7). Any dispassionate historian would agree. Without the pioneering work on anastomoses by Carrel, the early experiments on graft placement by Murray, together with the experimental trials with antirejection drugs, we would still today regard the diagnosis of CRF as a death sentence.

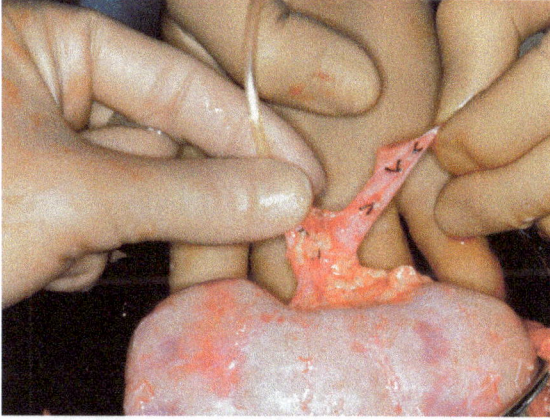

Fig. 9.5 A donor human kidney is perfused with saline prior to transplantation.

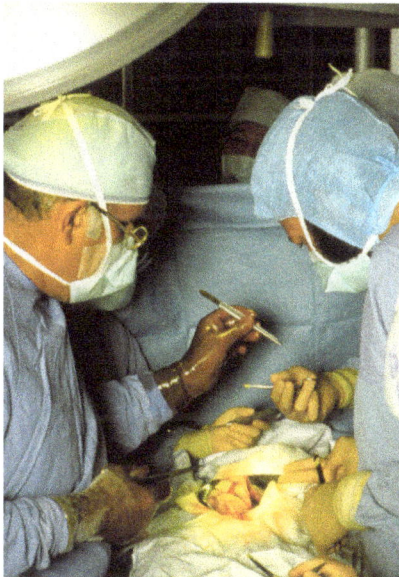

Fig. 9.6 Surgeons performing a kidney transplant operation. Of the 2,000 patients a year in the UK who receive a transplant, two thirds can expect their graft to survive for at least 10 years (Ref. 1).

Three Nobel Prizes have been awarded (Carrel in 1912, Medawar in 1960 and Murray in 1990) for work that has assisted in the success of transplantation. Many might argue that even more scientists in this field merit such recognition.

ANIMAL EXPERIMENTS AND KIDNEY TRANSPLANTATION

1902	Anastomosis of blood vessels	Dog, cat
1950	Autotransplantation of kidney	Dog, cat
	Perfection of placement surgery	Dog
1953	"Actively acquired tolerance"	Mouse
1955	Immunosuppressant effect of high dose radiation	Rabbit, dog
1959	Immunosuppressant drugs	Rabbit, dog
1963	Antilymphocyte serum	Mouse, rabbit, horse
1965	Tissue typing	Mouse
1989	New immunosuppressants, antibodies	Mouse, dog, monkey

An earlier version of this chapter was published as: The contribution of animal experiments to kidney transplantation. *RDS News* April 1995 8-14.

References

1) West R (1991) *Organ Transplantation*. London: Office of Health Economics.

2) Calne R (1970) *A Gift of Life: Observations on Organ Transplantation*. New York: Basic Books.

3) Carrel A (1902) La technique operatoire des anastomoses vasculaire et la transplantation des visceres. *Lyon Med* **98** 859.

4) Carrel A (1912) Technique and results of vascular anastomoses. *Surg Gynec Obst* **14** 246.

5) Carrel A (1910) Remote results of transplantation of the kidney and spleen. *J Exper Med* **12** 146.

6) Williamson C (1926) Further studies on the transplantation of the kidney. *J Urol* **16** 231.

7) Moore F (1964) *Give and Take: The Development of Tissue Transplantation*. New York: Saunders.

8) Little C & Tyzzer E (1916) Further experimental evidence on the inheritance of susceptibility to a transplantable tumour, carcinoma (JWA) of a Japanese Waltzing mouse. *J Exp Res* **33** 393.

9) Gorer P (1937) The genetic and antigenic basis of tumour transplantation. *J Path Bact* **44** 691.

10) Gibson T & Medawar P (1942) The fate of skin homografts in man. *J Anat* **77** 299

11) Murray J (1982) Reminiscences on renal transplantation, in Chatterjee S N (ed.) *Organ Transplantation*. Boston: John Wright.

12) Owen R (1945) Immunogenetic consequences of vascular anastomoses between bovine twins. *Science* **102** 400.

13) Lillie F (1916) The theory of the free martin. *Science* **43** 611.

14) Cannon J & Longmire W (1952) Studies of successful skin homographs in the chicken. *Ann surg* **135** 60.

15) Billingham R, Brent L & Medawar P (1953) "Actively acquired tolerance" of foreign cells. *Nature* **172** 603.

16) Calne R (1970) Dedication in *A Gift of Life. Observations on Organ Transplantation*. Aylesbury: MTP.

17) Dempster W, Lennox B & Boag J (1950) Prolongation of survival of skin homografts in the rabbit by irradiation of the host. *Brit J Exp Path* **31** 670.

18) Main J & Prehn R (1955) Successful skin homografts after administration of high dosage x-radiation and homologous bone marrow. *J Nat Cancer Inst* **15** 1023.

19) Mannick J, Lochte H, Ashley T & Ferrebee W (1959) A functioning kidney homotransplanted in the dog. *Surgery* **46** 821.

20) Schwartz R & Dameshek W (1959) Drug-induced immunological tolerance. *Nature* **183** 1682.

21) Schwartz R, Dameshek W & Donovan J (1960) The effects of 6-mercaptopurine on homograft reactions. *J Clin Invest* **39** 952.

22) Calne R (1960) The rejection of renal homografts inhibition in dogs by 6-mercaptopurine. *The Lancet* **1** 417.

23) Baker R, Gordon R, Huffer J & Miller G (1952) Experimental renal transplantation: 1. effect of nitrogen mustard, cortisone and splenectomy. *Arch Surg* **65** 702.

24) Woodruff H & Burg R (1986) The antibiotic explosion, in *Discoveries in Pharmacology* vol. 3 ed Parnham M & Bruinvels Amsterdam: J. Elsevier.

25) Metchnikoff E (1899) Etude sur la resorption des cellules. *Ann Inst Pasteur* **13** 737.

26) Woodruff M & Anderson (1963) Effect of lymphocyte depletion by thoracic duct fistula and administration of antilymphocyte serum on survival of skin homografts in rats. *Nature* **200** 702.

27) Brent L & Sells R (1989) Notes on the history of tissue and organ transplantation, in Chatterjee SN (ed.), *Organ Transplantation. Current Clinical and Immunological Concepts.* Boston: John Wright.

28) Maggon K (1994) Immunosuppressive gold rush and drug development. *Drug News and Perspectives* **7** 389.

10. Cardiopulmonary Bypass: Making Surgery on the Heart Possible

In the early seventeenth century William Harvey established that there is continuity between arteries and veins, and that the heart pumps blood through these vessels in a circular fashion. Harvey developed his hypothesis by observation of the relatively slowly beating hearts of cold blooded animals, such as snakes, rather than those of warm-blooded animals, which beat too fast to detect the pattern of their motion. In his use of further observational and quantitative techniques to substantiate his theory, Harvey manifested an exceptional intellect and imagination.

Even Harvey, however, could not have imagined the progress in the treatment of cardiovascular problems that was to occur in the following three-and-a-half centuries. Today, a patient's heart and lungs can be temporarily supplanted by a mechanical pump and oxygenator. The heart can be stopped for many hours, opened and subjected to intricate surgery, such as the replacement of a heart valve with a manufactured prosthesis or with animal tissue. At the end of the operation the repaired heart and the lungs are re-plumbed into the circulation where they resume their normal function.

This technique of open heart surgery involves opening the chest and the catheterisation of the great veins carrying the blood returning to the heart from the system. This deoxygenated, venous blood is collected in a reservoir, then passed through an oxygenator. The freshly oxygenated blood is pumped back into the arterial circulation through a convenient artery. Thus, an adequate supply of oxygenated blood is maintained to the vital organs. The heart and the lungs are therefore out of the circulation, having been "bypassed" by the mechanical pump, functioning as the heart, and the oxygenator, standing in for the lungs.

http://dx.doi.org/10.11647/OBP.0055.10

The heart is rendered quiescent and kept viable by cooling and by perfusion of the coronary arteries with a "cardioplegic" solution, which prevents the heart beating and also supplies the heart with requisite nutrients and electrolytes. The artificial heart-lung circuit is filled with blood of the same group or with a synthetic priming solution, and clotting is prevented within this extracorporeal circuit by the use of heparin. The sudden increase in apparent blood volume when the patient is connected to the extracorporeal circulation requires appropriate adjustment of anaesthetic level. Under these conditions the heart can be operated on for many hours. Even long and delicate procedures such as the replacement of a heart valve can be performed at a leisurely pace.

It is hardly imaginable that anyone could believe that a procedure of this complexity, with many potential difficulties, such as the development of lethal air or clot embolism, could have been achieved without many pilot experiments in relatively large mammals (Table 1). However, animal rights literature asserts that it is a "fiction" to say that open heart surgery depended on animal experiments (1).

ANIMAL EXPERIMENTS AND OPEN HEART SURGERY

1916-35	Discovery and purification of heparin	Dog, pig, ox
1933-53	Development of extracorporeal technique Pumps and oxygenators	Cat, dog
1955-85	Elective cardiac arrest and preservation of the ischaemic myocardium	Dog, rabbit, rats

Early Experiments

The first use of cardiopulmonary bypass in a patient was by Gibbon in 1953. However, Gibbon had started experimental work on the technique 19 years previously. As is frequently the case, a particular clinical experience prompted Gibbon to consider this possible surgical innovation. In 1930 one of his patients died because of obstruction of the pulmonary artery with a massive embolus. This naturally provoked the thought that the blockage could have been successfully removed, and her life preserved, if even a portion of the patient's circulation could have been taken over by an extracorporeal heart and lungs (2), thus bypassing the obstruction in the pulmonary artery.

It was 4 years before Gibbon and his wife had the opportunity to test this technique in the Surgical Research Laboratories of the Massachusetts General Hospital. They found, to their surprise and delight, that it was possible to take over part of the pulmonary circulation of the cat by an artificial, extracorporeal circuit for four hours, with the cardiorespiratory function being adequately maintained (3). Repetition of the experiments under sterile conditions demonstrated that substitution of the heart and lungs of a cat for 20 minutes by mechanical devices was followed by recovery and survival for more than 250 days in 3 out of 13 animals. The remainder survived for between 1-23 days. In control experiments, simple occlusion of the pulmonary artery for 3½ minutes, with no bypass, produced permanent cerebral damage. Death always followed a 6½ minute occlusion (4).

During these early experiments on cats, Gibbon tested various types of pump and oxygenator. It was established that a pulsatile flow (such as occurs with the heart) was not essential for the proper functioning of the perfused organs. This meant that a comparatively simple roller pump could be used as a mechanical heart (perhaps surprisingly, roller pumps were found not to cause excessive breakdown of red blood cells). The oxygenator originally used by Gibbon was a rapidly moving hollow cylinder constantly gassed with a 95% oxygen, 5% carbon dioxide mixture. The withdrawn venous blood was trickled against the inner surface of the cylinder where it was spread into a thin film by centrifugal force. Oxygenated blood was collected at the bottom of the cylinder from which it was pumped back into the animal. Gibbon opted for this method of oxygenation since, unlike other techniques, it did not cause undesirable frothing.

Gibbon also established that, contrary to belief, large arteries (such as the femoral) could be catheterised and ligated, for the return of the blood to the circulation, without compromising the tissue normally served by the artery (2).

Refining the Technique

There was a hiatus in research from 1939-1945. Gibbon and others then began extensive experiments in dogs to perfect a technique whereby complicated and time-consuming operations could be performed inside the chambers of the heart, without the problems associated with complete occlusion of the vessels carrying blood back to the heart.

In a comprehensive paper, Gibbon described a series of experiments in dogs to test whether exclusion of the heart and lungs from the circulation and prolonged passage of the blood through an artificial lung would have any deleterious effect (5). Initial experiments merely involved passing venous blood through the pump and cylinder oxygenator for 80-180 minutes, with no occlusion of the vena cava. This experiment was simply to see if the passage of the blood through the extracorporeal circulation for a prolonged period produced any ill effects. These animals lived less than 12 hours, dying in coma. *Post mortem* examination showed that death was caused by multiple small clots throughout all the organs. Further experiments demonstrated that the lungs could filter out these microemboli under some conditions, but attempts to pass the blood through the lungs prior to its return to the entire system proved abortive.

Gibbon therefore included a metal filter into the extracorporeal circuit (300 x 300 micron mesh, thread thickness 140 micron). The apparatus including the filter was then used in 6 dogs for $2^{1/2}$ hour periods. All 6 dogs recovered rapidly after the operation and no haemolysis was induced by the filter. The animals were sacrificed between 42 and 106 days after the operation.

No sign of any infarction or damage was seen at autopsy. One of the dogs was observed to have but one kidney, yet even this animal had recovered with no renal complication.

Armed with the experience of these pilot experiments, Gibbon and his co-workers embarked on full scale heart and lung bypass experiments with the whole of the blood returning to the heart being passed through the extracorporeal apparatus for up to 113 minutes. In initial experiments the mortality in the dogs was 60%, death being due to haemorrhage or anoxia. More sparing use of the anticoagulant, heparin, and the administration of carefully chosen amounts of its antagonist protamine at the conclusion of the bypass reduced the haemorrhage. The apparatus was modified to enable the withdrawal of greater amounts of blood from the vena cava. Oxygen saturation of the blood was improved by placement of wire mesh over the surface of the rotating drum, this prevented filming and promoted greater exposure of the blood to oxygen. These modifications resulted in complete recovery of most animals. A few deaths occurred due to pericardial effusion.

The next step was to actually open the heart during bypass. Gibbon and co-workers carried out experiments on 29 dogs in which the septum between the atria was pierced under direct vision through the opened auricle. In 24 of these dogs the septal defect was then closed. Fourteen of these dogs survived and the defect became completely healed and covered in endothelium on both sides (6).

Air entering the heart and hence the coronary circulation whilst the heart was opened was a frequent cause of death during these experiments. However, in 12 experiments a small plastic cannula was placed in the left ventricle *via* a stab wound. Suction was continuously applied to this cannula, thus any air entering the ventricle was removed. Air embolism of the coronary arteries did not occur in any of these experiments (6).

The First Use of Cardiopulmonary Bypass in Patients

Thus, twenty years of experimentation enabled the considerable problems associated with the development of an artificial heart and lung machine to be exposed and progressively solved. By the early 1950s the mortality in experimental animals was down to 12%.

Gibbon was ready to perform the first open heart operations on patients, aided by the heart-lung machine, in 1952-53. The first was on a 15-month-old baby with severe congestive heart failure (7). The cause of the condition was thought by the referral physicians to be a hole in the interatrial septum. When the atrium was opened however, no septal defect was found. The baby died soon after the operation and the post mortem revealed a huge patent ductus arteriosus. Sadly, this defect could easily have been corrected had it been looked for during the operation (Fig. 10.1).

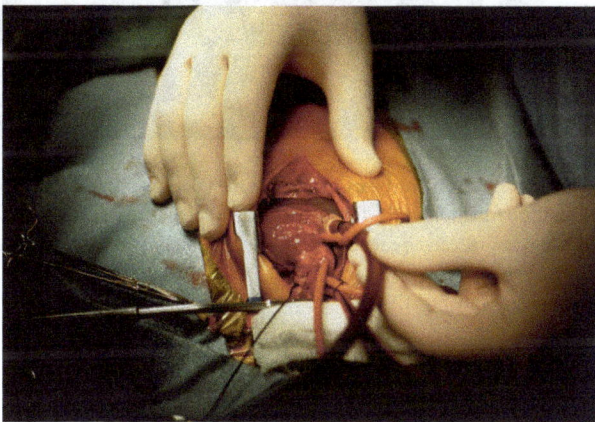

Fig. 10.1 The recently transplanted heart of a baby boy, showing the tubing still connecting it to the heart-lung machine. The donor heart was preserved by injecting it with chilled cardioplegic solution. © Science Photo Library, all rights reserved.

The second operation was performed on 6 May 1953. The patient was an 18-year-old girl who, although symptomless until December, 1952, had at that time developed right heart failure. Cardiac catheterisation revealed an atrial septal defect.

The patient was connected to the heart-lung circuit for 45 minutes during which time the heart was opened and the septal defect closed with a silk suture (7). The patient made a complete recovery and was alive and well at least 5 years later (2; Fig. 10.2).

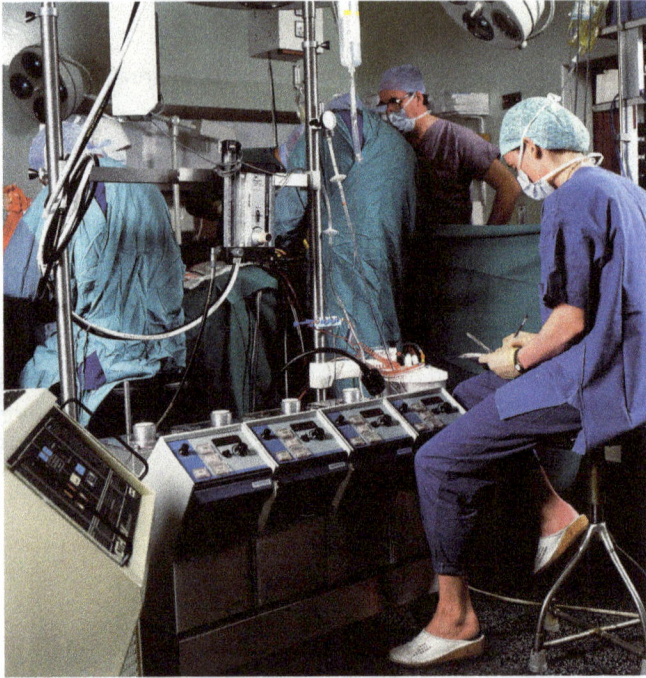

Fig. 10.2 In open heart surgery the heart-lung machine takes over the function of the heart with a pump and the function of the lungs with an oxygenator. This means that surgery, often taking several hours, can be carried out in relative safety to replace diseased arteries or defective valves. © Science Photo Library, all rights reserved.

Elective Cardiac Arrest

During the early open heart operations the flow of blood to the heart muscle continued through the coronary vessels. The persistent leakage of blood into the heart chambers from the coronary circulation necessitated the constant removal of this blood by suction, in order to maintain a clear field. The heart continued to beat, providing another hindrance to the cardiac surgeon.

In order to enable the operator to achieve the goal of "the unhurried correction of cardiac abnormalities under direct vision" (8), experiments were made to see if it was possible to stop and restart the heart at will, at the same time ensuring that no damage occurred to the heart muscle.

Melrose and his colleagues (8) achieved "elective cardiac arrest" in anaesthetised dogs on a heart-lung machine. Potassium citrate solution infused into the heart caused arrest within 5 seconds. After a token operation, blood was allowed back into the coronary vessels. Upon reperfusion with blood the hearts frequently went into ventricular fibrillation. Restoration of normal rhythm with a defibrillator was only possible in 70% of the experiments.

These researchers therefore performed further experiments on isolated, perfused hearts of rabbits to determine the optimal concentration of potassium necessary to stop the heart, and the allowable duration of the period of arrest. They concluded that potassium ions could be used to stop the heart pumping during bypass operations, and that hearts could recover spontaneously after 15 minutes arrest without becoming damaged. They also demonstrated that administration of calcium salts or adrenaline to restore heart beat was not only unnecessary but dangerous (adrenaline had frequently been used in the clinical setting to restart an arrested heart).

The Development of Cardioplegic Solutions

During the following decade the problems associated with ischaemia produced in the arrested heart were investigated and gradually solved. This was achieved almost entirely by studies on the rat heart.

One of the most important factors in the prevention of damage to the ischaemic heart is to stop the heart as rapidly as possible. High magnesium, zero calcium, acetylcholine, neostigmine and tetrodotoxin were all investigated for their ability to produce rapid cardiac arrest (9). Raised potassium concentration was found to be the method of choice, although preservation of the heart was found to be better with the chloride salt, rather than the citrate used by Melrose and his colleagues. Citrate had some toxic effect possibly due to chelation of calcium.

In a series of painstaking, carefully controlled studies lasting several years, Hearse and his colleagues at St Thomas's Hospital developed a cardioplegic solution that enabled hearts to be safely subjected to ischaemic periods of 4-5 hours. Their technique was simple. Rat hearts from freshly killed animals were perfused in an *in vitro* circuit. The hearts were subject to a 30 minute period of ischaemic arrest at 37°C. The post-ischaemic recovery of function (expressed as a percentage of the pre-ischaemic activity) was only 3%, indicating severe and irreversible myocardial injury. However, prior perfusion of the coronary vessels with a solution of potassium chloride (to stop the heart) caused a 10-fold improvement in recovery (i.e. to 30% of control).

Continuing with this technique, Hearse and his colleagues altered the concentration of various ions and other compounds within the cardioplegic solution (Fig. 10. 3).

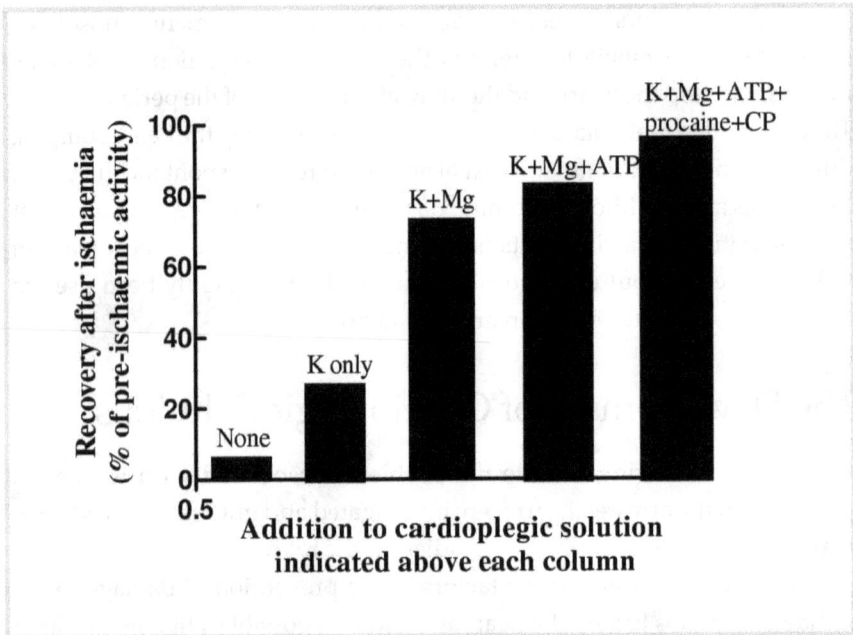

Fig. 10.3 Effect of additives on recovery of rat heart from ischemia. Data from D. Hearse (1988), 'The protection of the ischaemic myocardium: surgical success v clinical failure?', *Progress in Cardiovascular Diseases*, 30, 6, 381. The graph shows the beneficial effects of sequential addition of protective agents to cardioplegic solution. The protective solution was infused before a 30-min period of ischaemia of the isolated perfused rat heart. Without cardiac arrest the hearts only recovered 3% of their pre-ischaemic activity. With the progressive addition of various ions and chemicals recovery reached over 90%. Concentrations (mmol/L): potassium (K, 16); magnesium (Mg, 16); adenosine triphosphate (ATP, 10); creatine phosphate (CP, 10); procaine (7.4).

Surprisingly, it became clear that myocardial protection during ischaemia was not merely a matter of potassium arrest, for major differences in protection existed between solutions only slightly different in formulation. Ultimately the cardiac function, following even prolonged periods of ischaemic arrest, was restored to more than 90% of pre-ischaemic levels by the infusion of cardioplegic solutions of optimal composition prior to the ischaemia. Reducing the temperature of the solution to below 28°C ("cold cardioplegia") produced even greater improvement (10; Fig. 10.4).

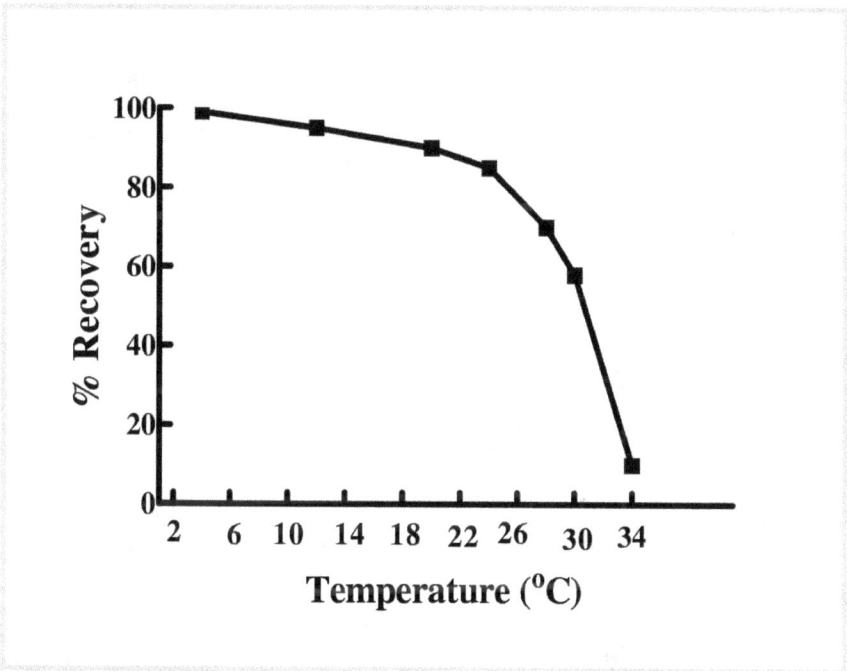

Fig. 10.4 Hypothermia and ischaemic injury. Data from Hearse (1988). The graph shows the beneficial effects of hypothermia on the ischaemic heart. Rat hearts were subjected to 60 minutes of ischaemia at various temperatures. Their recovery was measured 15 minutes after the end of the ischaemic period and expressed as a percentage of the activity before ischaemia. Hypothermia produced good protection if the temperature was kept below 24°C.

Further experiments, usually upon isolated, perfused rat hearts, have investigated the increase in efficacy produced by the inclusion of other chemicals in the standard cardioplegic solutions. Creatine phosphate, adenosine triphosphate, glucose, glutamate, aspartate, calcium antagonist drugs, procaine, glucocorticoids and many other substances have been shown to produce some degree of enhanced protection of the ischaemic myocardium in experimental studies.

Cold cardioplegia is routinely used in cardiopulmonary bypass operations throughout the world. Over 30,000 such procedures are carried out in the UK each year, with under 5% mortality. The "St Thomas' Hospital No. 1 solution" is almost exclusively used in the UK and widely used in Europe. In the USA St Thomas' solution No. 2 (*Plegisol*) is approved by the FDA (11; Table 2).

ST THOMAS' HOSPITAL CARDIOPLEGIC SOLUTIONS.
From Ledingham, Braimbridge & Hearse 1987 *J Thorac Cardiovasc Surg* **93** 240.

Composition (mmol/L)	Solution No 1	Solution No 2
Sodium chloride	144	110
Potassium chloride	20	16
Magnesium chloride	16	16
Calcium chloride	2.4	1.2
Sodium bicarbonate	--	10
Procaine hydrochloride	1	--

Cardioplegic solutions have also been used to preserve hearts prior to transplantation. With such a technique hearts have been successfully preserved for periods in excess of 15 hours (10).

The normal crystalloid cardioplegic solutions in present use, when cooled, provide good intraoperative protection for most patients. Clinical evaluation of solutions with various concentrations of the additives mentioned above will ultimately provide the best cardioplegic solution even for the high risk patient.

An earlier version of this chapter was published as: Cardiopulmonary bypass – making surgery on the heart possible. *RDS News* July 1995 8-12.

References

1) British Anti-vivisection Association (London) (1995) Pamphlet: Lies, damned lies ... and vivisection.

2) Gibbon J H (1959) Extracorporeal maintenance of cardiorespiratory functions. *Harvey Lectures* **53** 186.

3) Gibbon J H (1937) Artificial maintenance of the circulation during experimental occlusion of the pulmonary artery. *Arch Surg* **34** 1105.

4) Gibbon J H (1939) The maintenance of life during the experimental occlusion of the pulmonary artery followed by survival. *Surg Gyn Obst* **69** 602.

5) Stokes T L & Gibbon J H (1950) Experimental maintenance of life by a mechanical heart and lung during occlusion of the venae cavae followed by survival. *Surg Gyn Obst* **91** 138.

6) Miller B J, Gibbon J H, Greco V F, Smith B A, Cohn C and Allbritten F F (1953) The production and repair of interatrial septal defects under direct vision with the assistance of an extracorporeal pump-oxygenator circuit. *J Thor Surg* **26** 598.

7) Gibbon J H (1954) Application of a mechanical heart and lung apparatus to cardiac surgery. *Minnesota Med* **37** 171.

8) Melrose D G, Dreyer B, Bentall H and Baker J B E (1955) Elective cardiac arrest. *The Lancet* **ii** 21.

9) Hearse D (1980) Cardioplegia: the protection of the myocardium during open heart surgery: a review. *J Physiol Paris* **76** 751.

10) Hearse D (1988) The protection of the ischaemic myocardium: surgical success v clinical failure? *Prog Cardiovasc Dis* **30** 381.

11) Ledingham S (1992) Intraoperative myocardial protection, in P H Kay ed., *Techniques in Extracorporeal Circulation* 3rd ed. Oxford and Boston: Butterworth-Heinemann.

11. Artificial Heart Valves: From Caged Ball to Bioprosthesis

The heart is a dual pump. The right side receives blood from the body into the right atrium. From this chamber it passes to the right ventricle, a muscular pump capable of driving the de-oxygenated blood through the lungs *via* the pulmonary artery.

Freshly-oxygenated blood returns to the left side of the pump *via* the pulmonary vein. From the left atrium blood passes into the left ventricle, an organ powerful enough to pump blood through all the organs of the body.

The heart therefore pumps by a reciprocal mechanism. Blood enters a chamber *via* one orifice, then is pumped out through another. This means that valves are necessary to ensure that flow continues in the desired direction. Thus when the ventricles are contracting to direct blood to the lungs or to the general circulation, valves between the atria and ventricles are closed by pressure. This ensures that flow is directed through the pulmonary artery or the aorta. When the ventricles stop contracting, regurgitation of the blood back into the heart is prevented by valves that close the openings of these vessels (Fig. 11.1).

Valvular Defects

The cardiac valves are amazingly effective. They are flexible, economical on space, delicate in design yet remarkably strong. They survive great fluctuations of pressure every second throughout life and ensure a unidirectional flow of blood through the heart. It is therefore not surprising that if heart valves are affected by disease quite severe pathology ensues.

Lack of adequate patency of a valve (stenosis) or valvular incompetence can be due to congenital malformation, infection or atheromatous changes.

http://dx.doi.org/10.11647/OBP.0055.11

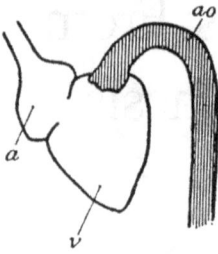

Diagram of a healthy heart in diastole. The aorta is full of blood under pressure. The ventricle and auricle are protected from the pressure by the aortic valve.

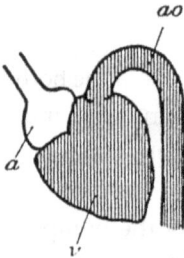

Heart with incompetent aortic valves. The ventricle, as well as the aorta, is under pressure during diastole. The auricle is protected by the auriculo-ventricular valves (mitral and tricuspid).

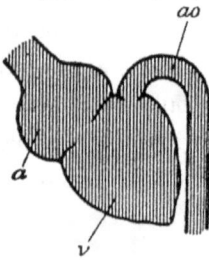

A heart with incompetent aortic and mitral valves. The auricle, veins, ventricle and aorta are all under pressure.

Fig. 11.1 Diagrams from: 'On Breathlessness, especially in relation to cardiac disease?' An address given by Lauder Brunton to the Willesden and District Medical Society and published in *The Practitioner* in June, 1905. Image in the public domain.

The pathology produced is that expected when an abnormal load is imposed on a chamber of the heart, or a back pressure created through the lung circulation.

Thus if the aperture of the mitral valve is narrowed, the left atrium and right ventricle bear the brunt of the defect. Both become enlarged (hypertrophied) and dilated. If regurgitation occurs, due to valvular incompetence, then the left ventricle will be involved and it too will hypertrophy. The pulmonary circulation may become engorged, with dilatation of the vessels, thickening of the alveolar walls and reduced oxygen transfer.

With serious defect of the mitral valve, death could be due to a variety of causes; maybe congestive heart failure, or cerebral embolism from a thrombus arising in a fibrillating atrium.

Similarly, in aortic valve disease, regurgitation results in gross enlargement of the heart (even to a weight of 1kg) with left ventricular hypertrophy and compensatory dilatation. Stenosis will produce a slowly developing hypertrophy. A patient with aortic valve disease will be prone to dizziness and fainting and will most likely die from congestive heart failure.

Damage to the tricuspid will tend to oppose the return of the blood to the heart, whereas defects of the pulmonary aortic valve will cause hypertrophy of the right ventricle (Fig. 11.1).

Treatment for Valvular Disease

Before the 1950s there was little one could do for serious valvular disease once it was established. In 1832 Corrigan stated: "cure of inadequacy of the aortic valve is probably beyond the reach of medicine" (1).

Even much later, White in his 1951 treatise (2) suggested nothing further than to advise the patient *"to protect himself against strenuous exertion or fatigue."*[1]

The development of the cardiopulmonary bypass technique, together with cardioplegia (see Chapter 10) provided a completely new outlook for the patient with valvular disease. The ability to open the heart and operate within it for perhaps hours, raised the possibility that defective heart valves could be excised and replaced with artificial substitutes.

Artificial Heart Valves: Early Designs

Natural heart valves are exquisitely designed. The mitral, for example, consists of two flaps of tissue, the free margins of which are anchored to the floor of the ventricle by thin strands of connective tissue called *chordae tendineae*. It offers virtually no impedance to the flow of blood into the left ventricle, yet prevents completely blood being forced back into the left atrium during the powerful contraction of the ventricle that sends blood throughout the system. It is an extremely effective valve yet takes up little space, being thin, pliable but totally unyielding to the pressures it is designed to resist.

It is not surprising that the earliest attempts to design a prosthetic valve tried to mimic the anatomy of the mitral valve with artificial materials.

One of the most intensive investigations was carried out at the University of Minnesota Medical School (3). The remarkable strength of cardiac valves is due to their collagen content. The team at Minnesota digested the valves of cattle and human cadavers with a proteolytic ferment that removed all protein except collagen. This enabled them to study the distribution of collagen fibres and their orientation along lines of stress.

Armed with this information, they manufactured valves from *Silastic* rubber-coated *Teflon* or *Dacron* felt. Imitation *chordae tendineae* were prepared by braiding strands of the felt prior to applying the rubber coating. It would of course be unthinkable to attempt to implant such a prosthesis into a patient without evidence that it could actually function. Therefore, as with all the various types of valve prostheses that were being made, they were put into dogs after excision of the mitral valve. The artificial flaps were sewn onto the mitral ring and the imitation *chordae* pulled through the wall of the heart and anchored outside at a suitable tension.

---

1   White did however refer to some palliative surgical interventions for some valve defects. For example, construction of an anastomosis between the aorta and pulmonary artery to ensure oxygenation of blood in severe stenosis of the pulmonary aortic valve.

This surgery was rather difficult. The prosthesis was emplaced successfully in only 7 out of 10 dogs. Only 2 of the 7 survived for a reasonable period (12 and 14 days). Small thrombi were observed on the atrial side of the prosthesis, particularly around the sutures.

It was soon realised that attempts to design a valve anchored by artificial *chordae* was going to be too difficult. If the *chordae* were made too long the valve flaps everted into the auricle, if too short, the valve was incompetent. Workers at the Mayo Clinic thus designed a "flexible cusp" valve (4). This, in essence, consisted of a firm plastic (*Mylar*) ring, to this was attached a thin, flexible sheet of plastic, strengthened by transverse "slats" of firm plastic. The flexible cusp was slightly larger than the ring, so that when forced against the ring by pressure it closed the orifice. The solid slats preventing the cusp being everted through the ring.

The comparatively simple design of the flexible cusp valve meant that the insertion of the prosthesis was relatively easy. Thus the dogs in whom it was tested were walking around within 5 hours of the operation and the valves appeared to function well initially. However the incessant movement and stress to which heart valves are subjected revealed the fragility of man-made materials compared to the archetype. Damage to the experimental valves occurred, in some cases as early as 5 days. Such poor durability precluded use in humans, where one would need to anticipate years of function.

Despite the disappointment of the lack of long-term success with these and the many other prostheses tested in the early 1960s, the experiments produced useful information. It was realised that for durability more robust materials were required. Thus the tendency for fatigue fracture was minimised by using woven material such as knitted *Teflon*. The increased durability resulted in increased post-operative survival, some dogs living for 72 days. The availability of even a few short-term survivors enabled the study of the anticipated problem of valve thrombosis.

Clot formation is bound to occur upon foreign surfaces, and within the heart or blood vessels where there is damage to the inner surfaces, for example where there are sutures. The workers at the Mayo Clinic noted that in their dogs clots tended to form at the suture lines then spread over the surface of the valve. The use of "non-irritant" suture, such as siliconised silk, or covering the sutures with *Ivalon* or natural valve tissue produced minimal benefit. Similarly, experiments with 9 different materials for the manufacture of the valve (including gold plated *Mylar*) had no significant effect on thrombosis formation. However it was established that valve design should ensure that there were no "nooks or crannies" where blood could stagnate and hence tend to clot (4).

There were many attempts to develop flexible, non-rigid artificial valves made of a wide variety of materials including, besides various compressed plastics and knitted *Teflon*, biological tissue such as pericardium and auricular wall. None was really reliable enough for human use.

There was undoubtedly a pressing clinical demand for an effective prosthetic valve. Eventually, it was realised that attempts to design a flexible prosthesis that would mimic faithfully the function of an endogenous valve would be abortive, at least without the advantages possessed by the original designer i.e. omniscience and unlimited time.

The Caged-Ball Valve

The cardiac surgeon Starr believed that one could not depend on the long-term flexibility of plastic materials emplaced in the heart, and opted for the development of a total replacement prosthesis that would not require extensive adjustment and manipulation in the theatre.

Starr developed a simple caged-ball valve (5). It consisted of a *Teflon* cloth ring to which is attached a lucite cage enclosing a *Silastic* ball. The ring was sewn into the mitral orifice of a dog, with the caged portion projecting into the ventricle. When the ventricle contracted the pressure increase forced the ball against the ring, effectively closing the orifice.

Compared to the other relatively delicate prototypes being tested at the time, Starr's ball valve must have seemed cumbersome, yet it was haemodynamically very good. The presence of the cage in the ventricle appeared to cause no damage to the inner surface, and contact between the cage and the ventricle wall produced no disorders of rhythm.

In Starr's first experiments, 80% of the dogs survived for at least 10 days, one was described as in "ferociously good health" 7 months after the operation (5) and later Starr reported survival continuing at 13 months (6).

The survival of these dogs enabled careful examination of the effectiveness of the valve by cardiac catheterisation (to measure left atrial pressure), angiocardiography and cine angiocardiography even 12 months after implantation. In some dogs steel pins were inserted into the *Silastic* balls so that valve function and ball spin could be observed with fluoroscopy.

Thrombosis was a serious complication with all valves tested in the dog so that evaluation of the long-term efficacy of valves had been difficult. Nevertheless with the caged-ball valve it was "possible to obtain long-term dog survivors without anticoagulant treatment" (7). This meant it was possible to establish the adequate functioning of the valve.

Encouraged by the experimental results, Starr performed mitral replacement in patients with a ball valve prosthesis from September 1960 (Fig. 11.2). This clinical work was published in October 1961 (7). By that time 12 patients had had mitral replacements. There were 2 post-operative deaths (not related to prosthesis) and 3 deaths from staphylococcal endocarditis (unfortunately there had been an epidemic of staphylococcal infection which eventually necessitated the closure of the operating suite). The remaining patients were well. The first 2 patients operated on were back at work. The Starr-Edwards caged-ball valve is still in use (8).

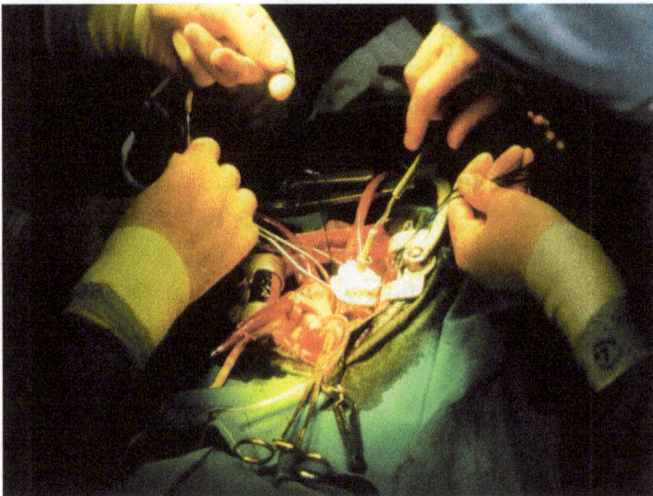

Fig. 11.2 Surgery to replace a mitral valve. Heart valve replacement surgery would not be possible without animal experimentation. The development of cardiopulmonary bypass techniques and cardioplegic solutions, necessary to carry out surgery on the heart, were explored in Chapter 10. © Science Photo Library, all rights reserved.

Refining Designs: Disc Valves

The relatively bulky construction of the caged-ball valve made it less suitable as a replacement for a defective aortic valve, particularly if the patient had narrow aortic roots. There was also the problem of the occlusion of the origins of the coronary vessels, which branch from the aorta just above the aortic valves.[2] So-called "low profile" valves were developed, such as a caged-disc

---

2   Actually, Hufnagel (17) had used a ball valve to combat aortic valve failure in 1951. Since this was before the development of cardio-pulmonary bypass techniques he implanted the valve in the descending aorta. Although not the ideal position, the prosthesis prevented 75% of the insufficiency and reduced the work load of the heart.

valve, which took up less room and would thus fit into the position of the aortic valve. This was not really an improvement for mitral replacement however, since the ball valve, having a freely rotating occluder, suffered less wear (Fig. 11.3).

The relative success of the caged-ball valve provided a boost to research on prosthetic valves. Engineering principles were used to study aspects of design that would provide maximum flow and minimal clotting. Davila and his colleagues from Temple University implanted many variations of suspended occluder valves in over 100 calves (9). They found that blood coagulation round the valve could be minimised by using highly polished surfaces on the prosthesis, hydraulic streamlining to reduce areas of stagnation or "wake" and graphite-benzalkonium-heparin coatings.

The design most favoured at present stems from the experiments of Wada, who implanted a tilting disc valve in the dog in 1964 and in man in the following year. The disc opened by a hinge mechanism which occasionally failed, resulting in fixation of the disc in the open position. Shiley designed an experimental valve with a freely rotating disc in 1968. Björk used a slightly modified design and evaluated it clinically in 1969. The Björk-Shiley valve is arguably the manufactured prosthesis of choice today (Figs. 11.4 and 11.5). Its simple design consists of a free-floating disc occluder suspended in a *Stellite* cage covered with a *Teflon* ring. The disc opens to 60° and closes between two eccentrically situated legs (10). As with all other synthetic prostheses however, some

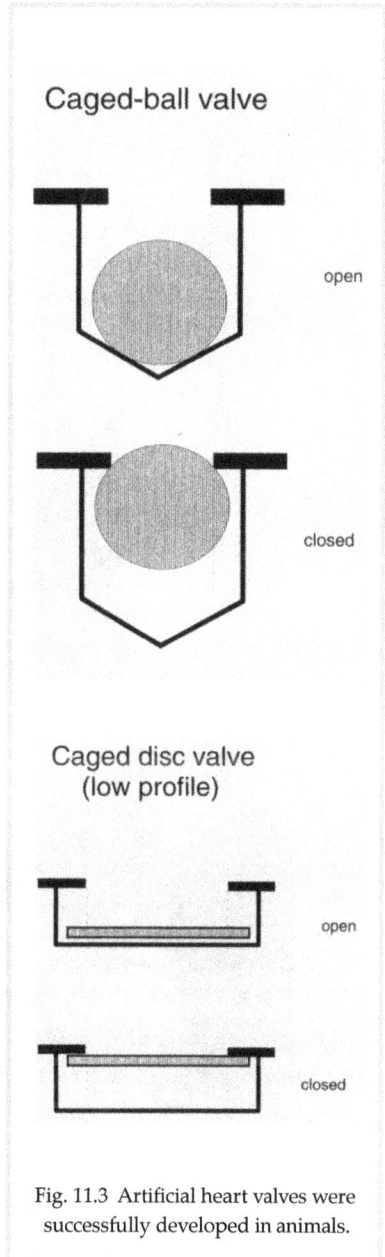

Caged-ball valve

open

closed

Caged disc valve (low profile)

open

closed

Fig. 11.3 Artificial heart valves were successfully developed in animals.

anticoagulant treatment is essential to prevent thrombosis. This is a distinct disadvantage of these devices, despite their proven efficacy over 30 years.

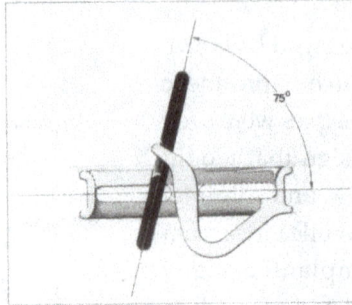

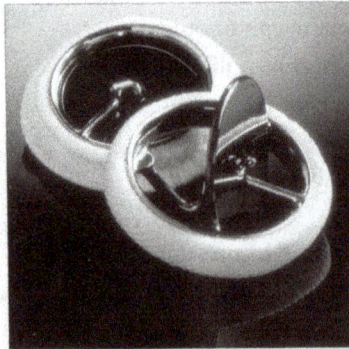

Fig. 11.4 The tilting disc aortic heart valve, with the tilting action shown in cross sectional profile. Picture courtesy of Medtronic, all rights reserved.

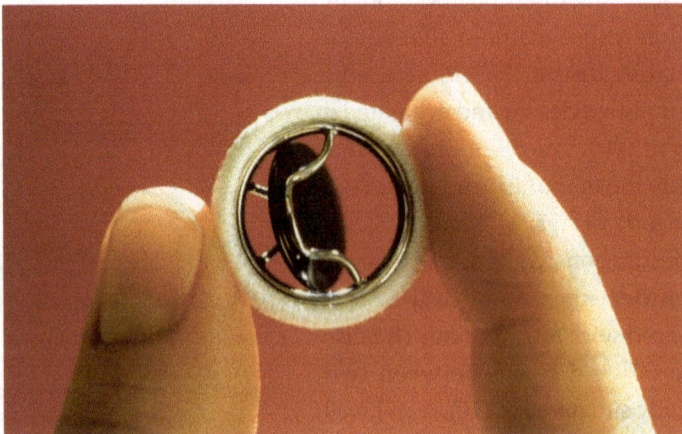

Fig. 11.5 Tilting disc aortic heart valve. © Science Photo Library, all rights reserved.

Allograft Valves

Carrel had shown that vascular tissue could be transplanted and arterial grafts had been used to counter various vascular defects. Until 1952 however, only cylindrical sections of blood vessels had been so transplanted. Stimulated by the success of the ball valve, implanted in the descending aorta, in the treatment of aortic valve insufficiency, Lam transplanted the aortic valve from a donor into the aorta of a recipient dog (11). The transplanted valves would function but only if the recipients own aortic valve was rendered incompetent by cutting one of the cusps. Of significance was the fact that there were no thrombotic complications. This allograft transplant technique was used in humans (12) in 1960 and later Duran and Gunning actually managed to place the donor valve in the natural, subcoronary position. Not surprisingly, the valves functioned well haemodynamically. The rejection complications that were experienced with these non-vascular, relatively inert pieces of tissue in many cases appeared to be minor. Therefore there were many experimental studies in dog to establish the optimal methods of preparation and storage of the valves before transplantation (13). With the limited techniques examined, the use of fresh tissue appeared best, although freeze drying or storage in betapropriolactone conferred some advantages.

Such studies began to subside when it became clear that there were severe logistic problems in the reliance upon the availability of sterile, allograft valves of the ideal size. By the mid-1960s it was realised that valves from other species would "solve all procurement and size problems if combined with a suitable sterilisation method" (13).

Transplantation of Animal Heart Valves: Xenografts

Freeze-dried pig aortic valves were placed into the aortae of dogs (14), some of which survived 8 months. Following this experiment there were many other studies where valves from pig, sheep, calf or goat were transplanted into other species, usually dog (15). Rejection phenomena were variable and were inhibited by azathioprine, although the use of long-term immunosuppressant therapy in patients was not considered a viable prospect. Significantly, there were no problems of clotting around the valve.

Research became focused on methods of treating the valves before transplantation to ensure durability and, by reducing antigenicity, prevent rejection. One of the most comprehensive studies was that of Carpentier and his colleagues (16). These workers made various extracts of xenograft valves and tested their antigenicity by agglutination tests in appropriately inoculated rabbits, intradermal tests in guinea pigs and immunofluorescent studies of differently treated valves implanted subcutaneously in rat. It was found that extensive washing or electrodialysis could remove much antigenic material, the remainder (mainly glycoprotein) was denatured by metaperiodate oxidation. The remaining free reactive groups on the valve were bonded together by a tanning agent, glutaraldehyde (this also prevents the subsequent denaturing of the collagen in the implanted valve, which would result in loss of shape and flexibility).

By this treatment Carpentier and his colleagues produced a biologically inert, functional and durable valve. After such treatment it could not accurately be termed a xenograft. Carpentier described it as a "bioprosthesis" – something between a graft and a synthetic prosthesis. Clinical experience with the bioprosthesis (usually porcine) has been good, with a negligible rate of thromboembolism.

Corrigan's quote: "cure of inadequacy of the aortic valve is probably beyond the reach of medicine" has been confuted. Today patients that develop serious valvular defects need no longer simply be advised to avoid "strenuous exertion or fatigue." With a prosthetic or bioprosthetic valve they can anticipate a decade symptom-free, possibly without the disadvantage of anticoagulant therapy. It is difficult to imagine that this could have been achieved without the animal experiments that began in 1933 with Gibbon's first attempt at cardiopulmonary bypass in cat.

Aanticoagulants for Prevention of Clotting Around Heart Valve Prosthesis

The foreign surfaces of artificial valves will inevitably initiate clotting. Anticoagulant therapy is thus essential for patients with valve prostheses. Although heparin (which is extracted from animal tissues) is a valuable anticoagulant that can be used temporarily after the immediate post-operative risk of haemorrhage, it is not orally active, and thus of no use for long-term anticoagulant therapy.

The standard anticoagulants used for prophylaxis with heart valves are all chemically similar to the prototype drug, *Warfarin*.

Warfarin was developed as a consequence of the study of a strange bleeding disorder that suddenly occurred in cattle on the northern prairies of the USA in the early years of the last century. Surgical procedures such as dehorning could result in fatal haemorrhage. In severe cases animals developed large haematomas and would bleed from the nose.

An astute veterinarian noted that the condition invariably followed the ingestion of hay or silage of sweet clover which had become spoiled during storage. Sweet clover had been planted on the comparatively poor soil of North Dakota at the end of the nineteenth century since it could be used as a substitute for corn for use as silage.

The isolation of the active anticoagulant from the "biochemical rag-bag" of the spoiled clover/hay was no easy task (18). An assay method had to be developed to track the effects of the "haemorrhagic agent" during the various extraction procedures. A measurement of the activity of the extracts on the prothrombin time, performed on diluted plasma from a particular strain of rabbit was ultimately chosen as the most suitable assay. After four years the active substance was identified as dicoumarol (3,3'-methylenebis(4-hydroxycoumarin)).

Many derivatives were synthesised, including *Warfarin*. These are used today to treat deep vein thrombosis as well as to limit the danger of thromboembolism in patients with synthetic valve replacements.

An earlier version of this chapter was published as: Artificial heart valves: from caged ball to bioprosthesis. *RDS News* October 1995 6-11.

References

1) Corrigan D (1832) On permanent patency of the mouth of the aorta, or inadequacy of the aortic valves. *Edinburgh Med & Surg J* **37** 225.

2) White P (1951) *Heart Disease*. 4th ed. Macmillan.

3) Schimert G et al. (1961) Fabrication of mitral leaflets and aortic cusps from Silastic rubber-coated Teflon felt, in *Prosthetic Valves for Cardiac Surgery* ed. Merendino K, Springfield: CC Thomas.

4) Frater R & Ellis L (1961) Problems in the development of a mitral-valve prosthesis, in Merendino, Ref. 3.

5) Starr A (1961) Discussion in Merendino, Ref. 3, p 319.

6) Starr A & Edwards M (1961) Mitral replacement: The shielded ball-valve prosthesis. *J Thoracic Cardiovasc Surg* **42** 673.

7) Starr A & Edwards M (1961) Mitral replacement: Clinical experience with a ball-valve prosthesis. *Ann Surg* **154** 726 (discussion p 740).

8) Vitale N et al. (1995) Long-term follow up of different models of mechanical and biological mitral prostheses. *Eur J Cardiothor Surg* **9** 181.

9) Davila J et al. (1967) Prosthetic cardiac valves: principles and problems, in Segal B & Kilpatrick D (eds.), *Engineering in the Practice of Medicine*. Baltimore: Williams & Wilkins.

10) Björk V & Henze A (1979) Prosthetic heart valve replacement. Nine years' experience with the Björk-Shiley tilting disc valve, in Ionescu M (ed.), *Tissue Heart Valves*. London: Butterworths.

11) Lam C, Aram H & Munnell E (1952) An experimental study of aortic valve homografts. *Surg Gyn Obst* **94** 129.

12) Murray G (1960) Aortic valve transplants. *Angiology* **11** 99.

13) Angell W, Pillsbury R & Shumway N (1969) Storage and function of the canine aortic valve homograft. *Arch Surg* **99** 92.

14) Duran C & Gunning A (1965) Heterologous Aortic Valve Transplantation in the Dog. *The Lancet* **ii** 114.

15) Paton B (1972) Experimental transplantation of aortic valves into desending aorta, in Ionescu M, Ross D & Wooler G. (eds.), *Biological Tissue in Heart Valve Replacement*. London: Butterworths.

16) Carpentier A et al. (1969) Biological factors affecting long-term results of valvular heterografts. *J Thoracic Cardiovasc Surg* **58** 467.

17) Hufnagel C (1951) Aortic plastic valvular prosthesis. *Bull Georgetown Univ Med Centr* **4** 128.

18) Beck E (1984) The treatment of thrombosis, in Parnham J & Bruinvels J. (eds.), *Discoveries in Pharmacology*, vol. 2. Amsterdam: Elsevier.

12. Animals and Blood Transfusion

Doctors misled for over 200 years:

History shows that a dependence on animal research delayed the introduction of blood transfusion by over 200 years.

NAVS Leaflet, Ever had a blood transfusion?

The assertion that animal experiments delayed the development of blood transfusion derives from the superficial and inaccurate accounts found in animal rights literature (see for example Ref. 1, page 157; Ref. 2 page 220). A brief review of primary sources reveals that animal experiments were crucial to the development of a) the concept of the benefit of blood transfusion, b) techniques for carrying out transfusion and c) the preservation of incoagulable blood and thus to the establishment of blood banks.

The function of the heart and the details of the circulation of the blood through arteries and veins were, of course, demonstrated by William Harvey in 1628. Harvey used about 50 species to elucidate the nature of the circulation. He studied, by means of a magnifying glass, the motion of the heart in "a small shrimp" found in the Thames (probably a species of mysid (3)). He obtained clear proof that the heart pumped blood *via* a closed circulation through arteries to the veins by simple experiments, using ligatures, on the slowly beating hearts of cold-blooded animals. In warm-blooded animals he could "neither rightly perceive at first when the systole and diastole took place, nor when and where dilatation and contraction occurred by reason of the rapidity of the motion, which in many animals is accomplished in the twinkling of an eye, coming and going like a flash of lightning" (4). Experiments on sheep, deer and dog demonstrated that the heart pumped in unit time a larger quantity of blood than is found in the whole body – thus clearly demonstrating a circulatory system.

http://dx.doi.org/10.11647/OBP.0055.12

By the early 17th century therefore, the concept that blood was pumped *via* the arteries to the organs was well established. To some observers at least, the blood began to be perceived not only as "the vehicle of the soul with the secrets of individuality" (5), but as a transporting system. It was therefore no surprise that experimenters should endeavour to infuse medicaments into the circulating blood of a living animal. Christopher Wren and Robert Boyle, in 1656, inserted a quill attached to a bladder (in later experiments, a syringe) into a superficial vein of a dog and successfully injected first opium, then the emetic, antimony oxide (5).

Early Transfusion Experiments

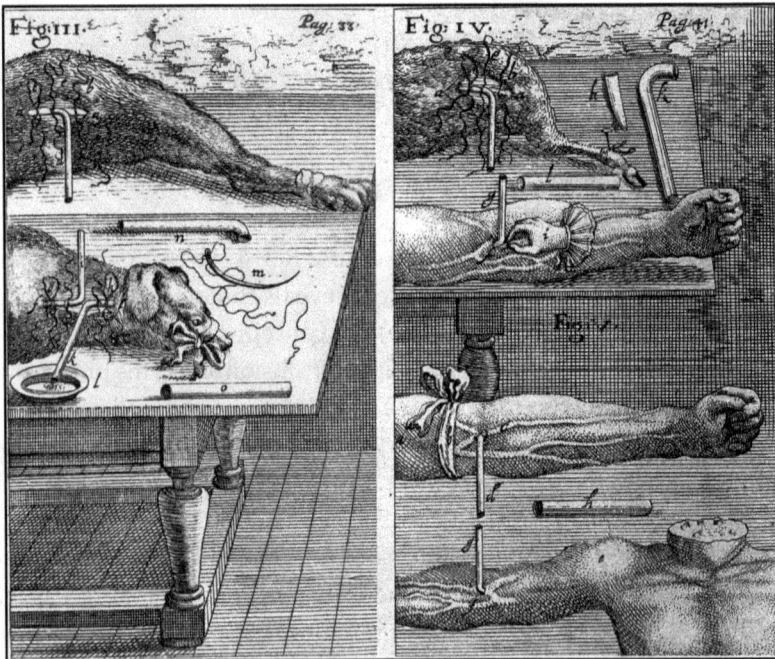

Figs. 12.1a and 12.1b Engraving showing transfusion in the neck and leg of a dog, from animal to man, and from man to man, by J. S. Elsholtz, 1667. Wellcome Library, London, CC BY.

This experiment doubtless led to attempts to transfuse blood from one animal to another. The earliest, well-authenticated account of the transfusion of blood from one dog to a second is that of Richard Lower, who in February 1665 used quills (and later a silver tube) to transfer blood from the carotid artery of one dog to the jugular vein of a second (6) (Fig. 12.1a). A later demonstration of the technique is described in Pepys's diary of November 14th 1666, where the recipient dog was described as "very well, and likely to do well." The diary also records subsequent discussion, which included musings as to the effect of transferring blood of a Quaker to an Archbishop. Boyle also queried whether the transfused dog would still recognise his master after receiving the strange blood (6). Thus although animal experiments had demonstrated the feasibility of transfusion, many still regarded the blood simply as the vehicle of the soul. The potential of the technique was clearly not appreciated.

The first person to transfer animal blood to a human was the French philosopher and mathematician Denis (spelt Denys in some accounts). With the help of the surgeon Emmerez Denis in 1666 allegedly transfered 9 ounces of blood from the carotid artery of a lamb into a 15 year old youth, moribund following excessive venesections to alleviate an obscure fever (Fig. 12.1b). Apparently, astonishing improvement resulted. Denis performed the operation on a further three subjects with no untoward effect, although the artery to vein anastomoses, with the chance of coagulation, made estimations of the amounts transfused dubious (Fig. 12.2).

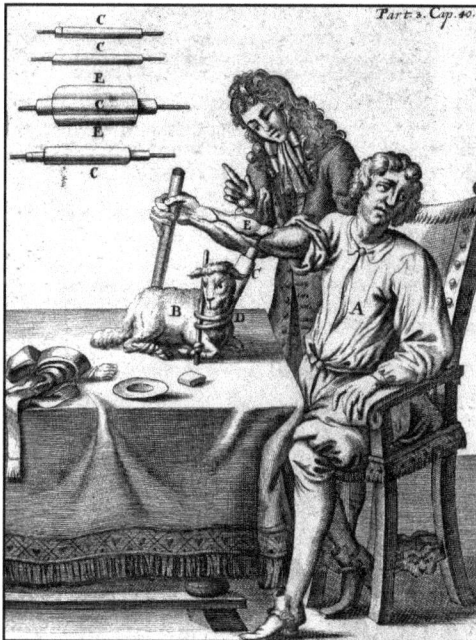

Fig. 12.2 Attempt at blood transfusion from lamb to man, depicted in an illustration dating from 1705. Wellcome Library, London, CC BY.

His last patient was a man "with an inveterate phrensy, occasioned by a disgrace he had received in some amours," presumably a gentle euphemism for neurosyphilis. Denis considered that calf's blood "by its mildness and freshness might allay the heat and ebulition of his blood" (7). The patient apparently tolerated two transfusions with some benefit upon his mental state, although the second was followed by pain in the kidneys and the production of black urine. At the behest of the patient's wife Denis attempted a third transfusion after which the patient died. Denis had enemies prominent in the Faculty of Medicine of Paris who were implacably opposed to transfusion of animal blood into man. He was charged with murder but eventually exonerated after counter charges that the patient had been poisoned by his wife. Nevertheless experiments on transfusion of blood into humans were prohibited by an edict of the French Parliament.

This official ban on transfusion in France is proposed by opponents of animal experiments as an argument that such techniques thus "delayed the practical availability of blood transfusions and led directly to the deaths of patients" (8). However, if transfusions between different species had been investigated before the transfusion of animal blood to man, the incompatibility of bloods of different animal species would have been established in the 17th century instead of 150 years later.

The efforts of 17th century opponents of transfusion to stigmatise the technique as evil and against nature probably worked for the best. Medicine and technology were not sufficiently advanced for doctors to use transfusion effectively. Knowledge of the function of the blood, of sepsis, of immunology and of clotting mechanisms were minimal or non-existent. Methods for transferring coagulable blood between individuals, without the benefit of materials available today, were fraught with problems and danger. It was therefore not surprising that during the 18th century references to transfusion were rare, and those described were irrational (in 1792 for example, Russell claimed to cure a child of rabies by injection of lamb's blood (6)).

Scientific Reasons for Transfusion

The gradual accumulation of physiological and pathological knowledge changed the perspective with which transfusion was viewed. Rosa and Scarpa (1788) recommended transfusion as a treatment for anaemia, and in 1796, Erasmus Darwin (grandfather of Charles) advocated tranfusion of blood in cancer of the oesophagus and other conditions resulting in inadequate nutrition. Darwin suggested transfusion could be effected *via* goose quills connected by a piece of chicken gut (6). There is no evidence that he attempted transfusion using this technique, but it is a salutary reminder of the primitive nature of the tools available for a complicated procedure.

Transfusion for Haemorrhage

Provost and Dumas in 1821 showed that animals haemorrhaged to the point of death could be revived by transfusion of blood, but not serum or water warmed to 38°C. Blood from animals of other species was not effective, since the animals appeared to survive but succumbed within a few days. Provost and Dumas did not attempt transfusion in humans, since they considered the basic knowledge of blood and its functions too rudimentary and, since the technique was too celebrated, it had already "been abused in an ignorant and barbarous century" (6).

Blood transfusion in humans was established as a sound scientific and clinical procedure by James Blundell (1790-1877), a lecturer in physiology and midwifery at the United Hospitals of St Thomas and Guy. Blundell was moved by the many deaths he had witnessed in patients with *post partum* haemorrhage. Even when bleeding had been suspended, frequently the patients had lost so much blood that one could do nothing but observe them sinking until death followed within 2-4 hours. In such cases, argued Blundell, "there is a fit opportunity for trying the operation of transfusion" (9).

In his extensive monograph (9) Blundell described his experiments in dogs that established that death from haemorrhage could be prevented by transfusion of blood from the same species, even if vital signs had been lost. Recovery occurred even if the volume of the blood transfused was a fraction of that lost (even just 20%). Transfusion of blood from another species was *not* effective, but venous blood was as effective as arterial blood, even if its transfusion was delayed or if it was passed through a syringe.

After his experiments in animals, Blundell took the giant step of attempting transfusion of human blood to patients with severe haemorrhage. He performed the operation 11 times, at first only as a last resort in patients who were clearly irrecoverable. As experience with the technique was gained it was used in appropriate, seriously ill patients quite successfully. A typical case was reported in *The Lancet* in 1828 (10). One and a half hours after delivery a woman collapsed with extreme prostration, "blanched and perfectly bloodless in appearance." It transpired she had been bleeding freely into the uterus, unknown to the physicians. Stimulants (brandy and port wine) were freely given to no avail. Blundell transfused 8 ounces of blood, and the patient "rallied and became in every respect much better." The patient made a full recovery and later commented that she had "felt as if *life* were infused into her body."

In view of the obvious difficulties associated with supplying blood by the direct connection of the donor's artery to the recipient's vein, Blundell developed apparatus that obviated the need to cannulate the vessel of the donor. Venous blood was allowed to collect into reservoirs from whence it was pumped by syringe or allowed to flow under gravity (Blundell's "impellor" and "gravitator"; Fig. 12.3a; Fig. 12.3b).

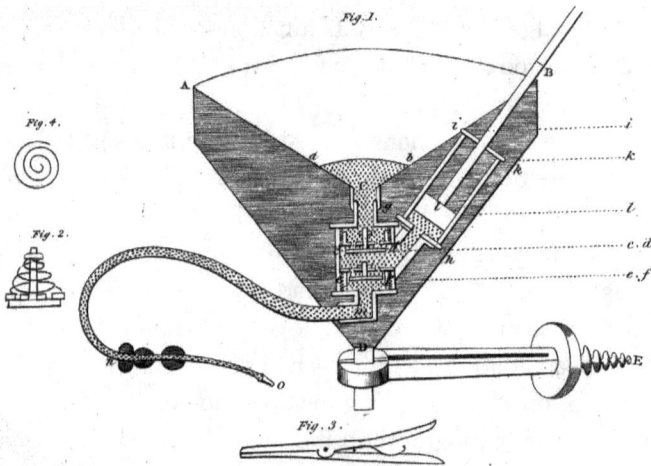

Fig. 12.3a Drawing of Blundell's impellor, which allowed venous blood to be collected in reservoirs before being pumped or allowed to flow under gravity to the recipient. (From Ref. 9). Wellcome Library, London, CC BY.

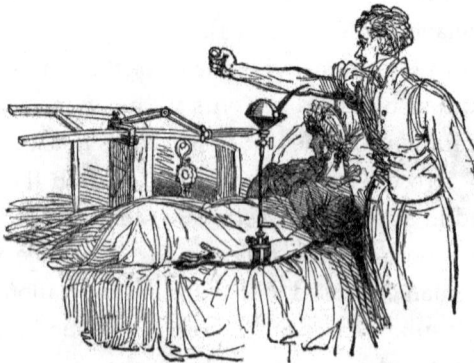

Fig. 12.3b Blundell's apparatus in use. From J. Blundell (1828). 'Observations on the transfusion of blood', *The Lancet*, 2, 321. Wellcome Library, London, CC BY.

Blood transfusion was thus established as a respectable and valuable procedure. It was not however commonly practised, but used as a last resort only. Some deaths still occurred even with human blood, but the real problem was simply the difficulty of carrying out such a formidable procedure. If reasonable volumes needed to be transfused, the clotting that was likely to occur meant that one had to transfuse by cannulation and connection of the artery of the donor to the vein of the recipient. This was certainly not a technique in which every physician was accomplished. It was not easy to persuade donors to have an artery cannulated and it was hard to regulate the amount transfused.

Landsteiner and the ABO Blood Group System

The necessity of transfusing blood of the same species, emphasised by Blundell, was reinforced by the observation by Crile (1869) that serum of different animals caused human red cells to clump. Landois (11) showed that animal serum caused actual lysis of human blood cells, thus explaining post transfusion haemoglobinaemia and the excretion of black urine in some early transfusions. These experiments definitively established that transfusion of animal blood to humans was absolutely contraindicated. It is thus surprising that even in the last quarter of the century some doctors, prompted by the lack of donors, were advocating transfusion of the blood of sheep.

The growth of immunology as a discipline provided clues to the reason for the incompatibility of human red cells with animal sera, since the lysis observed was considered analogous to the interaction of bacteria with antibody. Bordet found that the red cells of some species could generate antibodies in the plasma of another.

Prompted by earlier work, particularly that of Landois, Landsteiner was intrigued by the "biochemical species specificity" and considered "whether specific differentiation goes beyond the level of species, and also whether the individuals within a species show similar, though presumably slighter differences" (12). By mixing the serum and red cells of different human individuals Landsteiner established the ABO blood groups system. This obviously had great significance for the transfusion of compatible blood. Landsteiner's work explained the failure of some early transfusions. The successes of Blundell and others were presumably due to the fortuitous use of compatible donors and recipients.

Some transfusion reactions occurred even with matched samples in the ABO system. In the 1920s Landsteiner and Levine detected other agglutinins

(MN and P) in all four blood groups by injecting rabbits with human blood and showing the presence of raised antibodies to the human antigens (13).

Methods of Transfusion

Even though the matching of blood reduced transfusion reactions, at the start of the century the problem of clotting still prevented blood transfusion becoming routine. Blood clots when it comes in contact with any surface save the inner lining of blood vessels. Thus clots formed perhaps in the transfusion cannulae could enter the circulation and cause pulmonary embolism. For this reason transfusion was rarely performed, particularly when infusions of isotonic salt solutions became popular.

Carrel in 1902 (14) developed a technique in animals for joining arteries to veins, thus providing a continuous endothelial surface that enabled blood to flow from one vessel to the other without clot formation. This technique was put to practical use in a celebrated case that occurred a few years later, when Carrel was working as Research Fellow at the Rockefeller Institute. An infant of 5 days, suffering from haemorrhagic disease of the newborn, was bleeding from the nose and gut and was near death. The father, who was Professor of Surgery at Columbia University, knew of Carrel's experiments in anastomosing blood vessels of cats and dogs, and persuaded him to anastomose his own left radial artery to the child's right popliteal vein. The baby's colour changed from "white to pink and finally red all over." The infant stopped bleeding and made a complete recovery (7).

Carrel's technique was not simple, but Crile developed an easier method using a carefully constructed ring through which a vessel could be pushed and then everted over. The other vessel could then be pushed over the ring so that the intimal surfaces of the two vessels were thus in contact. A ligature around the ring secured the anastomosis. George Crile published this work in 1907 in the *Annals of Surgery*, stating that the paper "is based on 225 experiments upon animals and 32 clinical cases" (15).

Anticoagulants

By the early 1900s the prevention of blood coagulation was intensively investigated. Some delay in clotting was achieved by using paraffin wax-coated vessels to collect the shed blood prior to rapid transfusion *via* syringe. But what was obviously required was an innocuous substance that could be added to blood to prevent clotting. Some experimenters toyed with the use of the anticoagulant substance extracted from leeches, hirudin. Lewisohn (16) tested hirudin in dogs, one of which died. Nonetheless he decided to risk the administration of a small amount of hirudin to a patient who required a transfusion following a laparotomy for carcinoma of the stomach. The patient became cyanotic, had precordial pain, imperceptible pulse and was in a precarious position for 36 hours. This effectively removed hirudin as a candidate anticoagulant, although some workers used it to rinse syringes and vessels used in transfusion in the hope that clotting might be slowed.

The breakthrough came with the discovery that citrate could prevent clotting when added immediately to freshly collected blood, and that properly citrated blood was relatively non-toxic.

The distinction of being the first to advocate the use of citrate in blood transfusion is difficult to assign. The contenders are Hustin, Agote, Weil and Lewisohn. Most accounts accept that the Belgian, Hustin (17) was the first to infuse citrated blood to a patient. However, Lewisohn probably deserves the most credit since his careful experiments established the minimum concentration necessary to prevent clotting, and the amount of citrate likely to produce a toxic effect. In his classic paper (16) Lewisohn did however acknowledge "the priority, not only for taking up this problem in a series of animal experiments, but applying it successfully in a case of human blood transfusion, belongs to Hustin, though his method, as we shall see later, limited its usefulness to small transfusions."

Lewisohn added gradually increasing concentrations of citrate to 100 ml samples of dog's blood. He found that whereas 0.1% citrate had no effect, 0.2% and upward prevented clotting for days. Since 1,500 ml of blood might have to be transfused, Lewisohn obtained an estimate of the likely toxic dose. He withdrew 300 ml of blood from a dog, added increasing concentrations of citrate, and re-infused the blood. He found that a total of 1.5g of citrate in the blood was fatal for a dog of 11 lbs, suggesting that 15g would be toxic for a human of 110 lbs. Even an infusion of 1,500 ml of blood containing 0.2% citrate would thus be unlikely to be toxic to humans. Next Lewisohn investigated whether the infusion of citrate might lengthen the clotting time of the recipient's blood – certainly undesirable if the patient required a transfusion because of a haemorrhage. He found the coagulation time of blood taken from a dog was 5 minutes. He removed 300 ml of blood, added 0.2% citrate and reinfused. Samples of blood taken at 3 minute intervals after reinfusion were found, much to Lewisohn's surprise, to have a much *shortened* coagulation time (10 secs).

These careful experiments, and those of Weil, who showed that citrated blood could revive guinea pigs or dogs which had been practically exsanguinated (18), paved the way for the use of citrated blood for transfusions.

As transfusion became common practice, aspects of the toxicity of citrate needed to be reassessed. During exchange transfusion in neonates, for example, it was felt that toxic levels of citrate might be reached if the transfusion was too rapid. Experiments in dogs (19) showed that infusion of citrate at a rate of 0.06 mmol/kg/min was lethal, but 0.04mmol was safe. Rates of transfusion of citrated blood were therefore kept below 0.03 mmol/kg/min citrate, or where large volumes needed to be transfused, heparinised, rather than citrated blood was used.

Similar animal experiments alerted physicians to the possible danger of transfusing large volumes of blood that had been stored for a long period. Such blood tends to have high plasma potassium levels, since this ion leaks out of red blood cells in time. Infusions in rabbits showed that whereas the citrate or potassium in transfused blood produced only mild toxicity, a combination of both killed 15 out of a group of 19 rabbits (20). Thus the toxic effects of citrate and potassium reinforced one another. Where large volumes need to be transfused therefore (as in exchange transfusion in the newborn) fresh or heparinised blood should be used. Also, where patients have already high plasma potassium, for example anuric patients or those with extensive muscle wounds, only the use of fresh citrated blood is indicated.

Storage of Blood for Transfusion

Rous and Turner in 1916 (21) noted that there had been no investigation of methods to preserve the life of red blood cells *in vitro*, yet their improved preservation might have practical importance, even for transfusion. If stored in the cold for too long the cells tend to lyse. After a series of simple experiments on rabbit blood, Rous and Turner found that the addition of dextrose as well as citrate protected against lysis (Rous believed that since the cells are relatively impervious to sugars they would act like a colloid and preserve the cells. Subsequent research showed however, that the dextrose has a favorable effect on red cell metabolism). Blood so treated could be stored for 15 days and was still capable of reviving severely haemorraged rabbits, which unlike control, untransfused animals, survived and showed no anaemia. Blood cells stored longer than two weeks were still able to restore the level of haemoglobin in the bled animals, but in these cases the improvement was temporary, the animals becoming progressively anaemic.

These observations on the stabilisation of red cells were put to use in World War I at a US base hospital by Oswald Robertson (22), who set up the first (albeit limited) blood bank. Robertson, during periods of relative quiet, collected blood from universal donors (selected from patients with trivial wounds or those recovered from slight wounds) direct into dextrose/citrate and placed it in an ice box. Transfusions of the stored (10-14 days) blood were given to 20 patients, mostly haemorrhage cases. The results of these transfusions were "quite as striking as those seen after transfusion with blood freshly drawn."

The first recognised blood bank was set up in the 1930s at the Central Institute of Haematology and Blood Transfusion in Moscow. By 1937, 6,000 effective transfusions of stored blood had been made (7). The outbreak of World War II resulted in the establishment of transfusion services for the collection and storage of blood on a substantial scale.

Today, the storage and transfusion of sterile, compatible blood or blood constituents is a routine and life-saving procedure, the development of which depended upon the vision, experimentation and ingenuity of many physicians and scientists (Fig. 12.4). To suggest that blood transfusion was delayed for 200 years through dependence on animal experiments is totally incorrect. The implication of this assertion is that in 1714 transfusing coagulating blood through avian quills in non-sterile conditions could have been a routine procedure.

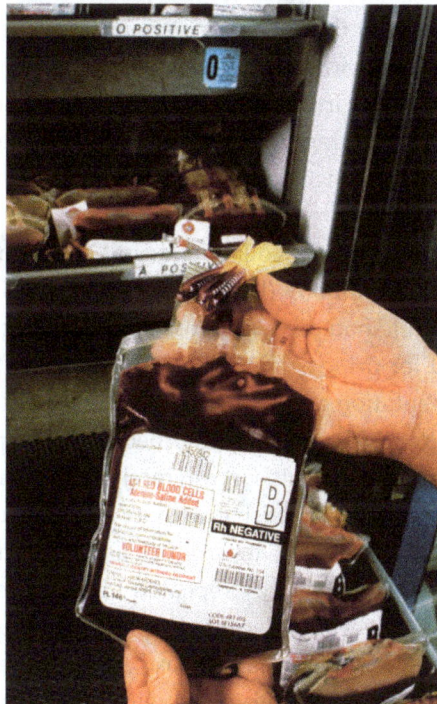

Fig. 12.4 Today, the storage and transfusion of sterile compatible blood or blood constituents is a routine and life saving procedure. © Science Photo Library, all rights reserved.

Such a denial of the contribution of animal experiments to human well-being stems from an unrealistic, facile conception of history.

Heparin

The potent anticoagulant heparin is not widely used to prevent the coagulation of blood to be transfused. It is, however, used for venous thrombosis and to prevent blood clotting during open heart surgery and kidney dialysis.

Heparin was discovered serendipitously in the liver of dog during a search for endogenous *clotting* substances (23). Heparin for clinical use must be obtained from pig intestine or bovine lung, and the crude extract is standardised by measurement of its anticoagulant action on sheep plasma (BP and USP).

The Rhesus Factor

Opponents of animal experiments have striven vigorously to establish that the rhesus (Rh) blood group system, despite its name, owes nothing to animal experiments. In fact it is difficult to establish who first discovered the Rh antigen. The history of this interesting scientific tale is well reviewed in Mollison (7). A reasonable interpretation is that Rh antigen was discovered in Landsteiner's laboratory in the early 1930s, by injection of rhesus monkey red cells into rabbits and guinea pigs, and adding their plasmas (containing anti-Rh antibodies) to human red cells. Landsteiner, however did not publish the work until 1940 (24).

Meanwhile Levine (a former collaborator of Landsteiner) together with Stetson, discovered an antibody (later shown to be anti-Rh) in the plasma of a woman whose child had died *in utero*. Since this work was published in 1939 (25), the credit for priority should go to Levine and Stetson. As far as the animal experimentation argument is concerned the question of priority is irrelevant. Levine and Stetson also described animal experiments in their paper, stating: "Agglutinins of this sort can rarely be investigated thoroughly because of their tendency to diminish in activity and eventually to disappear. Consequent attempts were made to produce a hetero-immune agglutinin of identical or similar specificity by repeated injections of sensitive blood into a series of rabbits. These experiments met with failure, since suitable absorption tests with such serums failed to reveal the presence of the desired agglutinin." Landsteiner, using rhesus red cells as antigen, was able to raise antibodies, which enabled the distribution of Rh group system in humans to be investigated.

THE DEVELOPMENT OF BLOOD TRANSFUSION

1628 Harvey	The circulation of the blood (about 40 species)
1656 Wren	Injection into vascular system (dog)
1665 Lower	Transfusion of blood between dogs
1666 Denis	Transfusion from lamb to man
1821 Provost and Dumas	Blood transfusion revived haemorrhaged animals
1824 Blundell	Must use blood of the same species for transfusion
1828 Blundell	Blood transfusion saved women dying from post partum haemorrhage
1869 Crile	Serum of animals causes human red cells to clump
1902 Landsteiner	ABO blood group system
1902 Carrel	Technique of anastamosis of blood vessels (cat and dog)
1915 Hustin and Lewisohn	Citrate safely used as an anticoagulant (dog and rabbit)
1916 Rous and Turner	With pre-treatment, blood stored for two weeks (rabbits)
1917 Robertson	Institution of blood banks for wounded soldiers
1933	First large blood bank established in Moscow

An earlier version of this chapter was published as: Animals and blood transfusion. *RDS News* July 1994 7-12.

References

1) Sharpe R (1988) *The Cruel Deception: The Use of Animals in Medical Research.* London: Thorsons.

2) Overell B (1993) *Animal Research Takes Lives.* NZ Antivivisection Society. Wellington, NZ.

3) Cole FJ (1957) Harvey's animals. *J Hist Med* **12** 106.

4) Lord Cohen (1957) ibid. 105.

5) Ficarra J (1949) Evolution of Blood Transfusion, in *Essays in Historical Medicine.* New York: Froben Press.

6) Zimmerman L & Howell K (1932) History of blood transfusion. *Ann Med History* **4** 415.

7) Mollison et al. (1987) Blood *Transfusion in Clinical Medicine,* 8th ed. Oxford: Blackwells.

8) Coleman V (1991) *Why Animal Experiments Must Stop.* Green Print.

9) Blundell J (1824) Some Remarks on the Operation of Transfusion, in *Physiological Researches.* London: E Cox & Son.

10) Blundell J (1828) *The Lancet* **ii** 431.

11) Landois L (1875) *Die Transfusion des Blutes.* Leipzig: Vogel.

12) Landsteiner K (1931) Individual differences in human blood. *Science* **73** 403.

13) Landsteiner K & Levine P (1927) Further observations on individual differences of human blood. *Proc Soc Exp Biol* (NY) **24** 941.

14) Carrel A (1902) *Lyon Med* **98** 862.

15) Crile G (1907) The technique of direct transfusion of blood. *Ann Surg* **46** 329.

16) Lewisohn R (1915) Blood transfusion by the citrate method. *Surg Gyn Obstet* **21** 37.

17) Hustin A (1914) Principe d'une nouvelle methode de transfusion. *J Med Brux* **2** 436.

18) Weil R (1915) Sodium citrate in the transfusion of blood. *JAMA* **64** 425.

19) Adams WE et al. (1944) The danger and prevention of citrate intoxication in massive transfusions of whole blood. *Ann Surg* **120** 656.

20) Taylor WC et al. (1961) Experimental observations on cardiac arrhytmia during exchange transfusion in rabbits. *J Pediat* **58** 470.

21) Rous P & Turner J (1916) The preservation of living red blood cells in vitro. I Methods of preservation. *J exp Med* **23** 219.

22) Robertson O (1918) Transfusion with preserved red blood cells. *BMJ* **i** 691.

23) Beck E (1984) The Treatment of Thrombosis, in Parnham M & Bruinvels J (eds.), *Discoveries in Pharmacology,* vol. 2. Amsterdam: Elsevier.

24) Landsteiner K & Weiner A (1940) An agglutinable factor in human blood recognized by immunosera in rhesus blood. *Proc Soc Exp Biol NY* **43** 223.

25) Levine P & Stetson R (1939) An unusual case of intra-group agglutination. *JAMA* **113** 126.

III. DRUGS FOR ORGANIC DISEASES

13. Animal Experiments and the Production of Insulin

Before 1922, the diagnosis of what was then called juvenile onset diabetes (type I or insulin-dependent diabetes, IDD), meant a lingering death within months. In that year, however, a team of workers in the physiological laboratories at the University of Toronto isolated and purified the hormone, insulin, from the pancreas. The purified insulin was shown to control not only the symptoms induced by removal of the pancreas in dogs, but also those of diabetes mellitus in patients.

The production of insulin on a large scale from pig and cattle pancreas was achieved fairly rapidly, due no doubt to the striking benefit that injection of insulin could produce in the seriously ill, even comatose, diabetic patient.

The effects of the ready availability of insulin were dramatic. This is illustrated by objective actuarial data produced by Metropolitan Life Insurance. This leading American insurance company stated: *"The results of this treatment have been brilliantly successful."* The data showed that the average age at death of diabetic patients in Toronto had increased by 22 years between 1920 and 1931. It also showed that: *"Deaths from diabetes among children under 20 years-of-age have almost ceased, and the death-rates under 50 years-of-age have declined very sharply."* (1).

The success of the Toronto team; Banting, Best, Macleod and Collip is rightly acclaimed by biomedical researchers as a prime example of undoubted benefit for patients achieved by animal experimentation. Presumably for this reason, the story of the discovery of insulin has been subjected to vehement attacks from animal rights adherents.

http://dx.doi.org/10.11647/OBP.0055.13

Early History of the Nature of Diabetes

Most physiologists accept that the observation of von Mering and Minkowski, that removal of the pancreas of dogs produced symptoms similar to those of patients with diabetes, was the crucial experiment linking the pancreas with the disease (2). Opponents of animal experiments claim that this observation was antedated[1] by significant work by Cawley, who in 1788 noted lesions in the pancreas of a diabetic patient at *post mortem* (3). Such an observation of course does not prove the lesions cause the disease, only that there may be an association between the disease and the observed damage. Changes in the blood vessels, kidney, retina and nerves also occur, but as a result rather than a cause of the condition. Nevertheless, antivivisectionists claim that Cawley's observation was a significant clue. They also imply that had this observation been followed up it could have provided a treatment for diabetes without recourse to animal experiments. Quite how this could have been achieved is not detailed by those who hold this view, and is not apparent to this writer.

Isolation and Purification of Insulin

By the end of the nineteenth century, the function of various glands was being investigated by their removal from animals and by examination of their extracts for physiological activity. Thus, adrenalin was extracted from the adrenal and thyroxin from the thyroid gland. It was therefore predictable that the then putative "antidiabetic" factor thought to be present in the islet cells of the pancreas should be designated "insulin" even before its successful isolation.[2] It was obvious at this time that insulin in some way enabled blood sugar to be properly utilised by the body.

The morbidity and mortality associated with diabetes ensured that there were immediate attempts to extract a factor (insulin) from the pancreas that could be used to treat this disease. This proved less easy than for adrenaline.

---

1 There is a claim that an exactly similar experiment to that of von Mering and Minkowski, demonstrating the appearance of diabetes in a depancreatised dog, was described in a book by Brunner in 1683, over 100 years before Cawley's observation (4).

2 Schafer apparently suggested this term in 1915. In some antivivisection propaganda, Schafer is implied to have discovered insulin in 1915, "six years before Banting and Best's experiments on dogs" (5). This is put forward as evidence against the contribution made by the Toronto workers, which is lauded by opponents of animal experimentation. (Adrenaline and thyroxine later acquired an 'e', presumably because they were eventually shown to be amines).

Minkowski tried, as did the French physiologist Gley, but probably the most important of the early studies was that of Zülzer (6). Zülzer used alcohol, rather than water, to extract insulin and he certainly produced active preparations. Forschbach, working in Minkowski's clinic in Breslau showed in 1909 that one of these extracts could reduce the blood sugar of depancreatized dogs by 90%. Unfortunately it also raised the temperature of the animal to 102.6°. Attempts to produce extracts of greater purity were made by chemists of the Schering Company, and these were given to two diabetic patients. The first produced no effect, the second caused a rise in temperature to 104° and the patient was unable to void urine for 12 hours. As a result of this toxicity the use of these extracts was abandoned in Europe at this time (7).

The Work in Toronto

Frederick Banting, a surgeon, and the medical student Charles Best began their attempts to prepare usable extracts of the pancreas in May 1921. Banting believed that it would be difficult to extract insulin, if it should be a protein, since during the process of extraction it would be bound to come in contact with protein-splitting enzymes which are also present in the pancreas. He therefore proposed ligating the pancreatic duct as a means of producing atrophy of the protease containing tissue. Extracts made from the pancreas so treated, Banting surmised, would have high insulin levels.

Banting's premise was in fact false on two counts (7). For this reason his published work came in for some criticism which has provided a focus for irrational condemnation of the work of Banting and Best and the role of animal experiments in the discovery of insulin (*vide infra*).

First, it is extremely unlikely that the pancreatic tissue could contain an active protease, since the active enzyme is only produced if its precursor comes in contact with the intestine. So there was no necessity to produce atrophy of the gland. Secondly, ligation of the pancreatic duct can also destroy the islet tissue. It was not therefore, as Banting and others believed, a technique that caused selective destruction of the acinar tissue.

Banting presented his first results at the New Haven meeting of the American Physiological Society in December, 1921 (Fig. 13.1). Extracts from both normal and "ligated" pancreas were shown to reduce blood sugar and abolish glycosuria in depancreatized dogs. The extracts had not been injected into patients. When this was tried a few weeks later the results were disappointing. The patients developed fever, and abscesses occurred at the injection site.

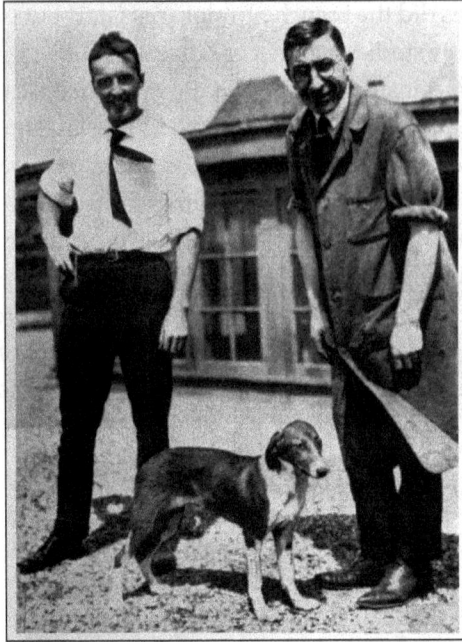

Fig. 13.1 The now famous picture of Frederick Banting, Charles Best and the dog Marjory, an early depancreatised dog treated with insulin, 1921. Wellcome Library, London, CC BY.

Non-Toxic Extracts

At this time Macleod, the head of the Physiology Department at Toronto, was persuaded to add a biochemist to the team to assist in the purification of the pancreatic extracts. This turned out to be a significant event. Within 2-3 weeks the biochemist, James Collip, prepared the first sample of insulin pure enough to treat diabetic patients from beef pancreas obtained from the slaughter house (7).

Collip used established techniques based on the selective solubility of different proteins in ethyl alcohol. This purification method required the measurement of the amount of insulin present in the various fractions produced. Since neither the nature nor the structure of insulin was known, the only way of assessing the amount of insulin present was by measuring its activity, i.e. by its ability to lower blood sugar levels in animals. Collip assessed the potency of each precipitate and filtrate in the process of fractional precipitation of the crude extracts by subcutaneous injection into fasted rabbits. One "unit" of insulin activity was described as that amount that would reduce the percentage blood sugar of a 2kg rabbit to 0.045 within four hours (8). The extracts prepared for clinical use were adjusted to contain one such unit in one millilitre. Thus animal experiments were absolutely crucial in the production of samples of insulin for the treatment of diabetes. An accurate method of standardisation of the extracts was essential. Even moderate overdosing with insulin can have serious consequences. Frank overdosing is lethal.

Clinical Success

The extracts prepared by Collip were used in dogs and patients with remarkable success (Fig. 13.2).

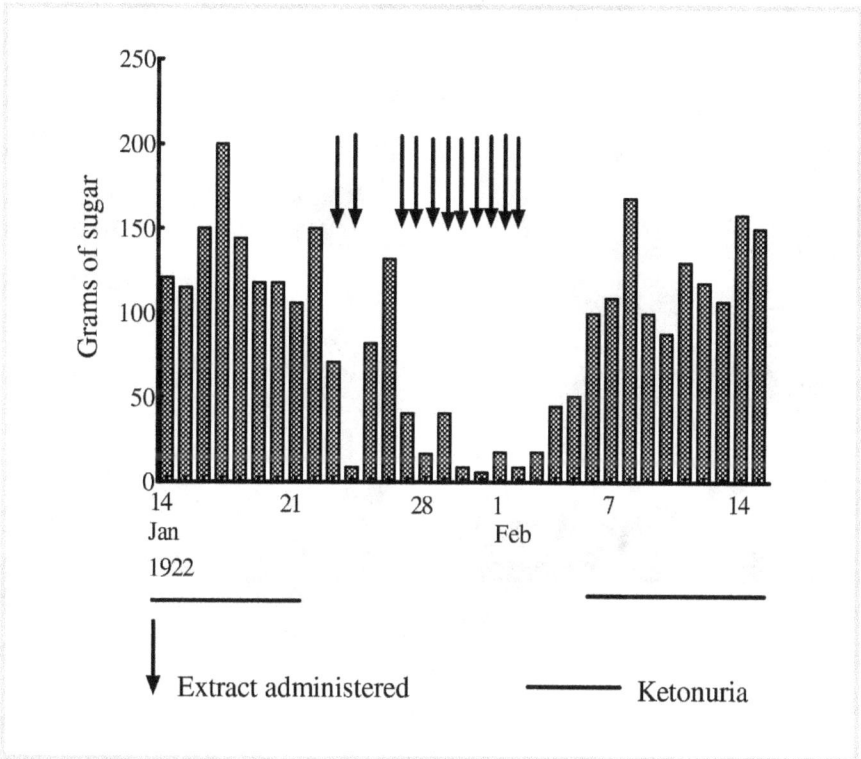

Fig. 13.2 The effect of Collip's highly-purified extract on the first patient to be successfully treated. Fourteen year old Leonard Thompson was given 10cc of the extract at 5pm on 23 January. The next day two injections of 10cc were administered. Sugar in the urine almost disappeared, ketonuria did disappear. Doses of 8cc of a new extract (presumably more potent) were given daily from 27 January onwards, markedly reducing sugar excretion in the urine. Data adapted from F. Banting, C. Best, J. Collip, et al. (1922), 'The effect produced on diabetes by extracts of pancreas.' *Transactions of the Association of American Physicians*, 1-11.

When the results of the Toronto team were reported at a meeting of the Association of American Physicians in May 1922, the distinguished diabetologist Dr Frederick Allen said:

> If, as seems to be the case, the Toronto workers have the internal secretion of the pancreas fairly free from the toxic material, they hold unquestionable priority for one of the greatest achievements of modern medicine (7).

Unless one has studied the case reports one can have no conception of the dramatic impact of the production of purified insulin. Diabetics placed on starvation diets, were reduced to emaciation and were barely able to hang on to a miserable life. With regular injections of insulin they could absorb and utilise a normal diet, gain weight, regain their vigour and flourish mentally and physically (Fig. 13.3).

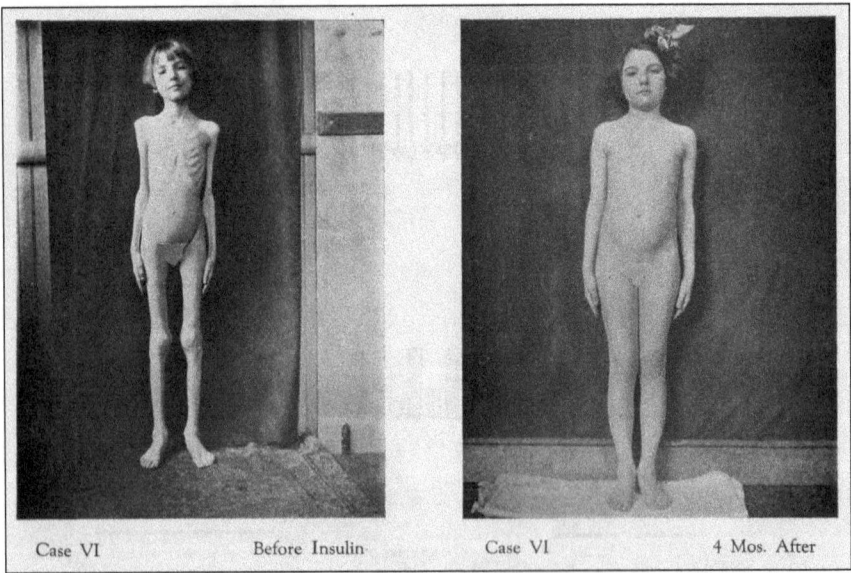

| Case VI | Before Insulin | Case VI | 4 Mos. After |

Fig. 13.3 Photographed in 1922, this diabetic girl, aged 13, weighed just 45lb before treatment with insulin. A few months later she had made a dramatic recovery.
Wellcome Library London, CC BY.

The Story of Elizabeth Hughes

A good example is that of Elizabeth Hughes. The daughter of an erstwhile Governor of New York State, she developed diabetes at the age of 11 years in 1918. Under the guidance of probably the best-known American diabetologist,

Dr Frederick Allen, she was placed on a restricted diet. Elizabeth became semi-invalid and was plagued by frequent infections. By 1922, although 5 feet tall she weighed under 50 lbs, only kept alive by her remarkable spirit and optimism. Elizabeth was taken to Banting's clinic in Toronto in August 1922. Banting's notes after his first examination of Elizabeth were:

> Weight 45 lbs. Height 5ft patient extremely emaciated, slight aedema of ankles, skin dry and scaly, hair brittle and thin, abdomen prominent, shoulders drooped, muscles extremely wasted, subcutaneous tissues almost completely absorbed. She was scarcely able to walk on account of weakness.

Banting placed Elizabeth on regular injections of insulin and, reasoning that she needed above all to put on weight, prescribed a liberal diet. For the first time for over three years Elizabeth ate bread, potato, macaroni cheese and also was allowed a daily pint of thick cream. She gained 10 lbs in 5 weeks, then gained a steady $2^{1/2}$ lbs per week. Elizabeth grew taller and, no longer restricted by her lack of energy to armchair activities, enjoyed trips to concerts, the cinema and even visited Niagara Falls.

In November 1922 the leading diabetologists of North America came to Toronto for a conference to discuss the initial clinical findings with insulin and to recommend methods for the standardisation of insulin dosage. Banting took a group of physicians, including Frederick Allen, to visit patients in his clinic. Allen did not recognise Elizabeth, and was rendered speechless by the healthy appearance of his former patient. Elizabeth (who was a compulsive and eloquent correspondent) described Allen's reaction in a letter to her mother: "Dr Allen said with his mouth wide open – Oh! – and that's all he did"

On November 30th, Thanksgiving Day, Elizabeth Hughes returned to her home in Washington. A year after graduating from college Elizabeth married. She raised three children and also in other ways led an active life, being an inveterate world traveller. On April 25th, 1981, almost 60 years after receiving her first dose of insulin, Elizabeth died of a heart attack (21). The discovery of insulin undoubtedly was *"one of the most dramatic achievements of modern medicine."*

Mixed Reactions

The familiarity that develops with passage of time obtunds the impact that a discovery such as the isolation of insulin had upon the medical profession and indeed upon the lay public. An effective way to get some sense of the reaction is to read contemporary comment in the general medical journals. A review of the research findings Banting reported at the May, 1922 meeting of the Association of American Physicians states:

> If these experimental observations prove clinically applicable to man clearly a magnificent contribution to the treatment of diabetes will have been made (9)

Other comments soon followed:

> Results which, it is not too sanguine to hope, have opened a new chapter in the history of the treatment of diabetes.

> As our readers have learnt from Professor Macleod, the effects observed in animals have justified the trial of insulin in man, and diabetic patients have eagerly flocked to take advantage of the new treatment (10).

> Readers ... cannot fail to draw the conclusion that a scientific advance of immense importance has already been accomplished (11).

As always, such approbation inevitably provoked some adverse criticism from the more conservative members of a markedly conservative profession. A particularly disparaging criticism appeared in the British Medical Journal on December 16th 1922. Dr Ff Roberts of the Department of Physiology, Cambridge University wrote:

> So much prominence has been given to the "insulin" treatment of diabetes that it is perhaps not out of place to review the steps which have led up to the production of this new remedy.

Roberts went on to assert that the hypothesis that ligation of the pancreatic duct would result in the destruction of the acinar tissue was incorrect, that in any case there was no need to attempt such an experiment for there is no active protease in the pancreas, and that Banting and Best's results clearly show that there was as much (or more) insulin activity in the "normal" as the "ligated" gland. Roberts concluded:

> The production of insulin originated in a wrongly conceived, wrongly conducted and wrongly interpreted series of experiments.

He conceded:

> apparent beneficial effects have been obtained in certain cases of human diabetes. Whether insulin will fulfil its promise time alone will show.

The next issue of the Journal (23 Dec, 1922) contained a letter from Henry Dale (later to become Sir Henry, Nobel Laureate) which was a devastating reproof of the "censorious criticism" by Roberts. Dale was at the National Institute of Medical Research in London, and was concerned with the standardisation by biological assay of the batches of insulin that were being prepared at that time. Dale's eloquent letter concludes:

> Nobody can deny that a discovery of first-rate importance has been made, and, if it proves to have resulted from a stumble into the right road, where it crossed the course laid down by a faulty conception, surely the case is not unique in the history of science. The world could afford to exchange a whole library of criticism for one such productive blunder, and it is a poor thing to attempt belittlement of a great achievement by scornful exposure of errors in its inception.

The ungraciousness of the comments by Roberts were also elegantly put into perspective by a leader that appeared in the British Medical Journal later:

> Dr Roberts' points are of a technical kind, and the terms in which they were expressed, it must be admitted, were wanting in *urbanity* (12).

The Criticism from Antivivisectionists

Despite the immediate condemnation of the somewhat ungenerous comments by Roberts, the quotation: "a wrongly conceived, wrongly conducted and wrongly interpreted series of experiments" continues to appear regularly in antivivisection literature and leaflets (5, 13), put forward as evidence that the public has been misled as to the value of the animal experiments of the Toronto group. This is quite wrong. Each of the Toronto team made an important contribution to the production of clinically useful insulin preparations. It was certainly the biochemist Collip who was responsible for producing extracts relatively free from toxic material, but as mentioned, the use of animals to monitor the purification of insulin was an absolutely essential part of this process. It is to be regretted that even advocates for moderate organisations supporting the development of alternative methods in medical research perpetuate the myth "that chemical extraction techniques (not involving animal tests) allowed the production of pure and safe insulin" (14).

Over half a century's experience has resulted in refinements in the use of insulin, particularly in the development of slow-release depot preparations to provide smooth therapy with the minimum number of injections. The miserable prospect for the IDD patient in the early 1920s is beyond the imagination of the lay public today, two generations divorced from direct anecdotal accounts. This public ignorance is utilised by antivivisectionists in their attempts to belittle the contribution of insulin to the treatment of diabetes. They assert that it is an *"absurd nonsense to claim diabetes has been cured"* since the number of people dying of diabetes has increased over the last 50 years and the number of diabetics is doubling every ten years (15). The fatuity of such arguments is patently obvious. They were summarily dismissed over 10 years ago by Rowan, who commented:

> These tactics are born of desperation. Since antivivisection protestors cannot deny that insulin therapy was derived from animal experimentation, the therapy itself is denigrated (16).

Insulin was never held to be a cure, it is merely a replacement therapy. Obviously, if diabetics treated with insulin can now survive for several decades rather than dying within a year or two of diagnosis, then the number of diabetic patients will increase. Even in insulin-treated diabetics the late complications of diabetes are often the ultimate cause of death. Thus deaths due to diabetes will appear to rise.

Another smoke screen raised by antivivisectionists is to introduce late onset diabetes (type 2 or non-insulin dependent diabetes, NIDD) into the equation. NIDD is of course more common than IDD and can often be treated by changing the diet. Thus antivivisectionists allege: "Today the great majority of diabetics who develop diabetes as adults control their disease through diet – they certainly do not need insulin injections." (15)

Stated in the context of discussion about the value of animal experimentation in the production of pure extracts of insulin, which is life-saving in IDD, this statement is wholly misleading. It can only be assumed that its intention is deliberately to misinform the public.

The Future

Human insulin can now be prepared by recombinant techniques. Physicochemical methods obviate the need for tedious bioassays of insulin extracts, no doubt to the considerable relief of those responsible for quality control.

However, administration of insulin by injection can never mimic the refined, minute by minute control of insulin release from the β-cells of the pancreatic islets, which is governed by plasma glucose levels. Thus diabetics are frequently hyper- or hypoglycaemic, with obvious pathological sequelae.

Transplantation of islet cells, which could release insulin as required, is an obvious answer once the problems of supply of cells and tissue rejection have been resolved. Porcine cells have been transplanted into nude mice and dogs. Rejection was prevented in the latter by antilymphocyte serum (raised in rabbit) and 15-deoxyspergualin. Such transplants have been attempted with some success in Swedish patients (17).

Another ingenious attempt to prevent rejection is the implantation of islet cells in capsules made of alginate. The capsule wall prevents access of host white cells to the islet tissue, but is sufficiently porous to allow passage of glucose and insulin. Exploratory experiments in diabetic dogs showed that a single treatment could replace injection of insulin for 6 months to 2 years (18).

Similar animal experiments will no doubt ultimately reveal the significance of the newly isolated compound "amylin." This peptide, which appears to be co-secreted from β-cells with insulin, increases blood sugar and is present in excess in NIDD (19).

Finally, a strain of mouse that naturally develops IDD (the non-obese diabetic [NOD] mouse) should eventually reveal the nature of the antigen that activates the immune system to destroy the islet cells of IDD patients (20). Even if the particular combination of genes that determine the genetic susceptibility to diabetes is established, a model such as the NOD mouse would be essential to establish the ultimate mechanism that triggers the destruction of the insulin-producing cells. Research with such models will set the scene for the prevention, rather than control, of IDD.

ANIMALS AND THE TREATMENT OF INSULIN DEPENDENT DIABETES

1889	Von Mering & Minkowski	Pancreatectomy produces diabetes mellitus (dog)
1900-22	Zülzer, Gley. Banting & Best	Pancreatic extracts lower blood sugar (dog)
1922	Banting, Best, Collip, Macleod	Extracts made from cows and pigs
1922-25	Banting et al.	Biological standardisation of extracts (rabbit, mouse)

An earlier version of this chapter was published as: Animal experiments and the production of insulin. *RDS News* January 1996 9-14.

References

1) Rogers R (1937) *The Truth About Vivisection*. London: Churchill, p. 109.

2) Von Mering J & Minkowski O (1889) Diabetes mellitus nach pankreas extirpation. *Archiv Exp Path Pharmak* **26** 371.

3) Sharpe R (1988) *The Cruel Deception: The Use of Animals in Medical Research*. London: Thorsons.

4) Yudkin J (1992) *New Scientist* 25 July, p. 51.

5) BAVA Leaflet (1995) Lies, damn lies and vivisection.

6) Bonta I (1983) Folklore, druglore and serendipity in pharmacology, in *Discoveries in Pharmacology*, vol. 1. ed Parnham M & Bruinvels J. Elsevier.

7) Pratt J H (1954) A reappraisal of researches leading to the discovery of insulin. *J Hist Med* **9** 281.

8) Macleod J (1922) Insulin and diabetes. *Brit Med J* **2** 833.

9) Anon (1922) Insulin and diabetes. *Brit Med J* **2** 140.

10) *Ibid.* p. 991.

11) *Ibid.* p. 882.

12) *Ibid.* p. 1233.

13) Overell B (1993) Animal Research Takes Lives. NZAVS.

14) Newman C (1994) Diabetes – what, why and how? *Alternative News* no 52 Dr Hadwen Trust.

15) Coleman V (1991) *Why Animal Experiments Must Stop*. London: Green Print.

16) Rowan A (1984) *Of Mice, Models, and Men*. SUNY Press.

17) Anon. (1995) Transplant of porcine pancreatic cells. *RDS NEWS* January, 1995.

18) Day S (1993) Jelly capsules offer end to diabetics daily dose *New Scientist* 4th September, 16.

19) Amiel S (1993) Amylin and diabetes. *The Lancet* **341** 1249.

20) Kaufman D et al. (1993) Spontaneous loss of T-cell tolerance to glutamic acid decarboxylase in murine insulin-dependent diabetes. *Nature* **366** 69.

21) Bliss M (1983) *The Discovery of Insulin*. Edinburgh: Paul Harris (All unreferenced items can be found in this outstanding historical account).

Acknowledgement: *Jack Botting acknowledges helpful discussions with Professor David Tomlinson.*

14. Animals and Humans: Remarkably Similar

The assertion that animal experimentation is a "failed technology" (1) is the linchpin of the pseudoscientific attack on animal-based biomedical research that has been waged over the last two decades. However, it is an undeniable fact that our knowledge of the function of the organs of the human body stems almost solely from research in other animals.

For example, the investigation of the function of the heart by William Harvey (2) was one of the earliest adventures in experimental medicine. Harvey's conclusion, that the movements of the heart caused the blood to circulate round the body, derived from observations in cold-blooded animals such as a living snake or toad as well as in the pig. Today, the rodent is the most widely used order for experimental work. It is evident that there is no difference in the way the conducting tissue in the heart of the rat or the human triggers the sequential contraction of the individual muscle fibres, so that the blood is caused to circulate first through the lungs then throughout the body.

The similarity extends to pathology, for should a coronary artery of the rat heart be ligated, thus preventing the flow of blood to a portion of the heart muscle, bursts of irregular heart beats occur – bigeminy, ventricular tachycardia – just as happens in patients suffering from acute myocardial ischaemia induced by coronary occlusion. Exactly as in patients, a proportion of rats so treated will die due to ventricular fibrillation unless resuscitation techniques are applied.

The mechanisms whereby the major organs are controlled and co-ordinated are likewise identical in man and laboratory species. The chemical messengers released from nerve cells in the brain and the peripheral nervous system to effect a response in adjacent cells are identical in all mammals. Thus,

http://dx.doi.org/10.11647/OBP.0055.14

for example, the increase in heart rate induced by circulating adrenaline or by noradrenaline released from sympathetic nerves in the heart can be blocked in both humans and rat by beta-adrenoceptor antagonists such as propranolol. Indeed even the selective blockade, by the more recent drugs, of the beta receptors on the heart as compared to those on the lung (preferred by asthmatics) is observed in the rat as well as man.

The more long-term regulation of organ activity of humans, that exerted by the endocrine system, is of course also analogous in laboratory animals. In fact in the absence of animal experimentation it is doubtful if knowledge of the functions of say, the pituitary and thyroid glands would be much different from the views current in the mid nineteenth century. At that time it was thought that they were concerned with the production of mucus to moisten the nasal and tracheal membranes respectively.

It is a fact that the hormones, insulin, obtained from the pancreases of pigs or cows, powdered thyroid gland of pig, thyrotropin obtained from cow pituitaries, calcitonin obtained from parathyroid glands of salmon, adrenocorticotrophic hormone from the pituitaries of "mammals used for food" and oxytocin and vasopressin from pig posterior pituitary glands have all been used in patients to correct hormone deficiencies or for diagnostic purposes. This surely speaks more powerfully for the similarity of the physiologies of these species rather than for patent differences.

One could of course fill a textbook with further evidence but these very general examples serve to illustrate the basic similarities in the physiology and biochemistry of all mammals and even non-mammalian species.

The Arguments

What are the arguments used by those attacking the validity of animal experiments? How do they attempt to justify their claims?

Diseases

First there is the claim that animals don't suffer from the same pathological conditions as man and therefore cannot be used to study human diseases which, it is alleged, are entirely different. In fact there are many animal diseases which are the exact analogy of those in humans. The veterinary surgeon Cornelius (3) has published a list of some 350 diseases suffered by animals which have an exact human counterpart. The paper of Cornelius is mentioned by the antivivisectionist Sharpe (4, p. 116) who quite erroneously claimed that Cornelius gives "a long list of animal *models* of human disease" (my emphasis), implying that these were induced, whereas in fact Cornelius was describing diseases that occurred spontaneously in animals. Cornelius went further to suggest that the study of such diseases was "a neglected medical resource" and called for coordinated interprofessional efforts between human and veterinary centres. This issue is also well-covered in a source readily available to the general public – the section on "Animal Disease" in *Encyclopaedia Britannica*. This contains a large list of diseases common to animals and humans and states: "it is likely that, for every known human disease, an identical or similar disease exists in at least one other species."

Reaction to drugs

The second argument is the claim that animals respond differently to drugs. It is often stated that there are vast differences between lethal doses in animals and humans (4, p. 98). The problems in making such a claim are clear. Whilst it is relatively easy on the one hand to obtain a satisfactory estimate of the range of toxicity of a substance in an animal species it is not possible in humans. One must rely on data from suicides or accidental poisoning where one can never be absolutely confident of the amount ingested or the amount possibly lost by vomiting or stomach wash etc. Furthermore, individual variation in humans due to genetic constitution, age (many cases of poisoning occur in children), alcoholism, concurrent ingestion of alcohol or other drugs, existing disease etc., render any but the most vague estimate of toxic dose impossible.

Similarly spurious are the claims of a particular drug morbidity produced in an animal species but not in humans. One of the most preposterous is the allegation by Sharpe (4, p. 72) that aspirin is a proven teratogen in rats and other species yet, despite being widely used by pregnant women has failed to produce any malformation. The studies in which aspirin was shown to be teratogenic in rat used doses of 250 mg/kg/day, from three days prior to mating to the end of pregnancy (5), or 300 mg/kg/day from the 9th to the 12th day of pregnancy (6). Transposed to the human (assuming a woman of 55kg) it would mean a regimen of 46 aspirin tablets per day for the whole of pregnancy or 55 tablets every day from the 12th to the 17th week of pregnancy (Fig. 14.1).

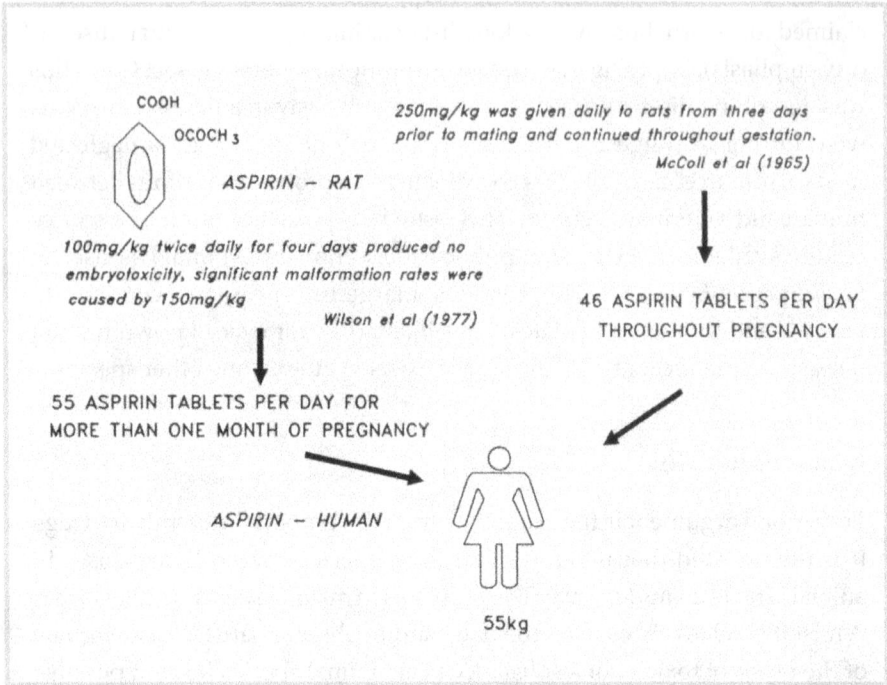

Fig. 14.1 Aspirin causes birth defects in rats, but not in people.

Not surprisingly, clinical data with this sort of regimen does not exist, however McNeil (7) cited 8 cases of fetal abnormalities in children from mothers who habitually took large doses of aspirin during pregnancy, and in a retrospective study by Richards (8) of 833 patients who ingested large amounts of aspirin during the first trimester, there was a significant rise in malformation.

One can similarly destroy the rather bizarre assertion that a hormone naturally produced by the body – insulin – "produces deformities in laboratory animals but not in people" (4, p. 72). In these studies (9) pregnant rabbits were given 20 units of insulin per day for between 2 and 13 days (a dose sufficient to cause hypoglycaemic convulsions for five hours each day) and many abnormal fetuses were born. Again, no comparable clinical data exists but one would hardly be surprised if pregnant women subjected to this treatment produced deformed children.

A final example is the perennial canard that morphine calms people but causes "maniacal excitement in cats" (4, p. 71). The source of this statement is obscure but the veterinarians Davis and Donnelly (10) showed that doses of morphine equivalent to those used in humans (i.e. 0.1 mg/kg) "produced analgesia with no excitement in experimental cats," and the current edition of a standard textbook of veterinary pharmacology (11) states: "Even in the cat, it is now accepted that very low doses (of morphine) can produce analgesia without excitement." A high dose of morphine (1 mg/kg) will produce excitement in cats, as it will in humans (12).

The flaws in the arguments raised by those proposing that animal experiments are "bad science" are easily exposed by reading primary sources readily obtainable in any science library. The selection and promulgation of abstracts that transmit a persuasive misrepresentation of scientific method does nothing for the furtherance of scientific or ethical principles.

An earlier version of this chapter was published as: Animals and humans – remarkably similar. *RDS News* January 1993 8-10.

References

1) Sharpe, R (1989) Animal Experiments – A Failed Technology, in *Animal Experimentation. The consensus Changes.* Oxford: Macmillan Press.

2) Harvey, W (1628) *An Anatomical Disputation Concerning the Movement of the Heart and Blood in Living Creatures.* Trans by Gweneth Whitteridge. 1976 London: Blackwell Scientific Publications.

3) Cornelius CE (1969) Animal models – A neglected medical resource. *New Eng J Med* **281** 934-43.

4) Sharpe R (1988) *The Cruel Deception: The Use of Animals in Medical Research.* London: Thorsons.

5) McColl J D, Globus M & Robinson S (1965) Effect of some therapeutic agents on the developing rat fetus. *Toxicol appl Pharmacol* **7** 409-17.

6) Wilson J G, Ritter E J, Scott W J & Fradkin R (1977) Comparative distribution and embryotoxicity of acetylsalicylic acid in pregnant rats and monkeys. *Toxicol appl Pharmacol* **41** 67-78.

7) McNeil J R (1973) The possible teratogenic effects of salicylates on the developing fetus. *Clin Paediat* **12** 347-50.

8) Richards I D G (1969) Congenital malformations and environmental influences in pregnancy. *Brit J Prevent & Soc Med* **23** 218-25.

9) Kalter H & Warkany J (1959) Experimental production of congenital malformations in mammals by metabolic procedure. *Physiol Rev* **39** 69-115.

10) Davis L E & Donnelly E J (1968) Analgesic drugs in the cat. *J Am Vet Med Ass* **153** 1161-67.

11) Brander et al. (1991) *Veterinary Applied Pharmacology and Therapeutics.* 5th ed. Philadelphia: Bailliere Tindall.

12) Goodman & Gilman (1980) *The Pharmacological Basis of Therapeutics.* 6th edition. New York: Macmillan.

15. Early Animal Experiments in Anaesthesia

In an attempt to make the history of scientific developments readable authors tend to highlight bizarre and amusing incidents, sometimes to the extent of inadvertently misleading the reader.

Thus most essays that purport to describe the background to the introduction of general anaesthesia to surgery inevitably refer to the laughing gas parties or ether frolics that were apparently commonplace in the 1840s (see (1) for example). The inhalation of nitrous oxide or ether produced instantaneous elation or inebriation. Social occasions where this activity was indulged were presumably more benign equivalents of today's glue sniffing sessions or Ecstasy parties. The conventional story is that accidental injury sustained during such a party was not noticed until well after the effects of the inhaled substance had worn off, suggesting to the astute observer that the apparent analgesic action of the inhalants might be of use in surgery. A good story, but is it true? The answer is only partially.

Fifty years before an anaesthetic was used in patients Humphrey Davy had demonstrated that nitrous oxide produced a state of unconsciousness in animals that was reversible if the animal was returned to air. He described the administration of nitrous oxide to a "stout and healthy cat" (2):

> after 5 minutes the pulse was hardly perceptible; he made no motions and appeared wholly senseless. After 5 minutes and a quarter he was taken out … in 8 or 9 minutes he was able to walk … in half an hour he was completely recovered.

Davy similarly described the effect of breathing a mixture of 1 part oxygen and 3 parts nitrous oxide on a guinea pig:

> … in 2 minutes reposed on his side, breathing very deeply … he lived quietly for near 14 minutes. He was taken out and recovered.

http://dx.doi.org/10.11647/OBP.0055.15

These experiments led Davy to conclude that animals could survive for long periods in an atmosphere of nitrous oxide mingled with air, and he subsequently inhaled the gas himself noting on one occasion that the gas relieved the pain caused by a wisdom tooth.

In his book *Researches* published in 1800 Davy concludes:

> As nitrous oxide in its extensive operation appears capable of destroying physical pain, it may probably be used with advantage during surgical operations in which no great effusion of blood takes place.

Henry Hickman, a practitioner at Ludlow in Shropshire, took the experiments a stage further by actually performing surgery on animals during a state of "suspended animation" induced by inhalation of carbon dioxide or nitrous oxide (3). As a result of his experiments Hickman tried to direct the attention of the medical profession in Britain (and later in France) towards the possibility of preventing pain during surgical operations by the inhalation of these gases (Fig. 15.1). However, his pamphlet: "A letter on Suspended Animation containing experiments showing that it may safely be employed during operations on animals with the view of ascertaining its probable utility in surgical operations on the Human Subject," appears to have been totally ignored by the Royal Society, before whom it was laid in 1823.

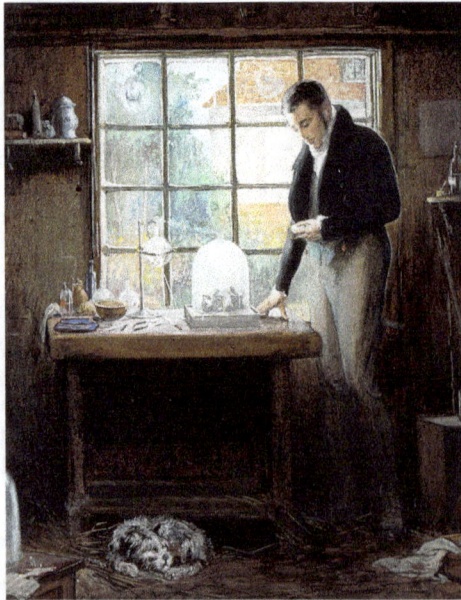

Fig. 15.1 Watercolour of Henry Hickman by Richard Cooper, painted in 1912. Hickman was a pioneer of anaesthesia, successfully performing surgery on animals anaesthetised with carbon dioxide as early as the 1820s. Wellcome Library, London, CC BY.

It was not until over 20 years later that the dentist Horace Wells, under nitrous oxide anaesthesia, had a wisdom tooth removed by his partner Riggs. The nitrous oxide was administered (at the behest of Wells) by Quincy Colton, a onetime medical student who made his living by demonstrating the effects of laughing gas on members of the audience at his stage shows. By 1846 major operations in both America and Britain were being performed under anaesthesia with ether, which Charles Jackson and Morton (an ex-partner of Wells) had found to produce a less erratic induction than the gas nitrous oxide, which only came into its own in 1868 when it was available compressed into cylinders. During the acrimonious dispute amongst the claimants that followed the announcement by the United States of a substantial prize for the inventor of anaesthetics, Jackson gave credit to Humphrey Davy when he wrote: "I have in former publications stated, as I do now, that my attention was first awakened to this subject while a student of medicine, by reading Davy's researches." (4)

It is clear that animal experiments paved the way towards the development of general anaesthetics and should have ensured their acceptance 50 years earlier but for societal reasons. The blossoming of humanitarianism and philanthropy that characterised the Victorian era fostered the desire to alleviate all suffering, even that of childbirth which was held to have authoritative support in the Book of Genesis.

It was the desire to find the perfect anaesthetic for the pain of childbirth that lead Simpson, the Professor of Midwifery at Edinburgh University, to search for an alternative to ether. Ether was not only an irritant but also inflammable, a risk when it was used in candlelight. Amongst other investigations he attempted to persuade Wemyss Reid to allow him to inhale ethylene dibromide, which had recently been prepared in the latter's laboratory. Wemyss Reid quite rightly insisted that the liquid should first be tested on rabbits. Two were subjected to the vapour, quickly passed into anaesthesia and in due course recovered. The following day Simpson intended to test ethylene dibromide on himself and his assistant but sensibly did not proceed with the experiment upon discovering that the two rabbits had died overnight (5) (ethylene dibromide is used today as a soil fumigant to destroy nematodes; it causes pulmonary congestion and depression of the central nervous system if inhaled). This was probably one of the earliest examples of the necessity of preliminary animal testing before phase one clinical studies.

Simpson eventually obtained a sample of chloroform (Fig. 15.2), a substance which had been tested on animals by Flourens and shown to produce unconsciousness (6).

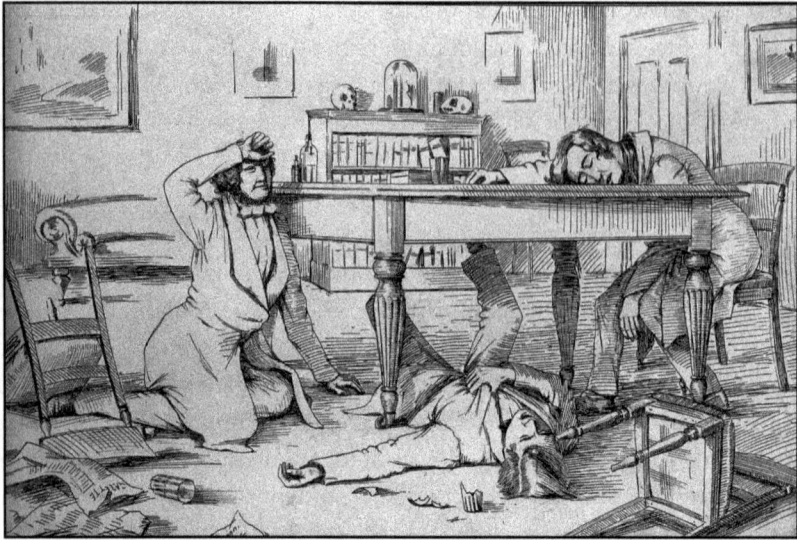

Fig. 15.2 Drawing of Sir James Young Simpson and friends by unknown artist, representing Simpson's discovery of the anaesthetic properties of chloroform in humans. Previously tested by Flourens on animals in the 1840s, chloroform was used almost immediately by Simpson to ease the pain of childbirth. Wellcome Library, London, CC BY.

Simpson used chloroform in midwifery and produced a paper describing its effects in November, 1847. As a result, chloroform rapidly came into use in general surgery and for a while was believed to be absolutely safe. However the first death under chloroform anaesthesia occurred two months later in January, 1848 (3) and there followed a high incidence of intraoperative and postoperative deaths due to the hepatotoxic and cardiotoxic actions of this anaesthetic. Animal rights propaganda, however, frequently avers that "chloroform is a useful anaesthetic for people, but poisonous to dogs." (7) Its dangers to patients are obvious but where is the evidence that it is inordinately toxic to dogs? Wakley in 1848 (8) compared the effects of ether and chloroform on 100 animals of various species. Out of 32 animals anaesthetised with ether, 11 died (34%). A total of 67 animals were given chloroform and 30 died (44%). Of the 17 dogs given chloroform only 4 died (24%). Hardly evidence for a selective toxic action.

It is clear that those who wish to promote the animal rights case on what are claimed as "scientific grounds," can carefully select the evidence they choose to transmit and so put forward an apparently plausible argument. However, omission of evidence can result in a misinterpretation of history. Whatever one considers the morality of a particular crusade, facts should be sacrosanct.

References

1) Sharpe R (1988) *The Cruel Deception: The Use of Animals in Medical Research.* London: Thorsons.

2) Livingston A (1983) in *Discoveries in Pharmacology* vol. 1 ed Parnham M J & Bruinvels J, Amsterdam: Elsevier.

3) Hewitt F (1912) *Anaesthetics and their Administration,* London: Macmillan & co.

4) Jackson C T (1861) *A Manual of Etherisation,* Boston: Mansfield.

5) Youngson A J (1979) *The Scientific Revolution in Victorian Medicine,* London: Croom Helm.

6) Flourens (1847). Note touchant l'action de l'ether sur les centres nerveux. *Comptes rendus* **24** 340-44.

7) NAVS Leaflet, Bitter Pills, The human consequences of testing drugs on animals.

8) Wakely T H (1848) One hundred experiments on animals, with ether and chloroform. *The Lancet* **i** 19.

An earlier version of this chapter was published as: Early animal experiments in anaesthesia. *RDS News* July 1992 4-5.

16. The Control of Malignant Hypertension

The reduction of the death and morbidity rates due to infective disease in the 1930s and 40s threw other pathological problems into sharper relief. Thus, in the developed world, cardiovascular disease and cancer became the major causes of death.

An important risk factor for many cardiovascular diseases is raised blood pressure, a symptom which the opponents of animal experiments imply could be avoided by changes in one's lifestyle – stopping smoking, taking exercise and reducing fat intake, alcohol and stress (see for example Ref. 1, p. 44). Even if one disregards the mutable nature of the evidence connecting diet with cardiovascular disease, and the undeniable contribution of one's genetic constitution to this condition, the implication that all cases of high blood pressure are so avoidable is certainly not in accord with clinical experience prior to the use of the first antihypertensive drugs.

Malignant Hypertension

High blood pressure accompanied by changes in the optic fundi (papilloedema) characterised a particular type of hypertension with a markedly rapid downhill course. Malignant hypertension, as it was known, could occur at virtually any age, and was generally fatal within one year of diagnosis. Contemporary clinical descriptions are to be found in the paper of Schottstaedt and Sokolow (2) who described the inexorable pathological progress of 104 patients aged from 13 to 71 years, who attended their outpatient department during the 1940s. The average survival time after discovery of papilloedema was 8.4 months. Initial symptoms were blurred vision and headaches. According to physicians treating the patients, the headaches could be devastatingly painful (3).

The difficulties of dealing with severe hypertension are described graphically by Dollery (4) in his admirable review of the history of hypertension treatments.

http://dx.doi.org/10.11647/OBP.0055.16

As a junior clinical student in the early 1950s he had to deal with a female patient admitted to an ear, nose and throat ward with nose bleed. She was found to have a very high blood pressure and papilloedema. After the bleeding was stopped she was "discharged on the grounds that the condition was untreatable." Dollery goes on to describe his subsequent experience (three years later) with the then current treatment of the most severe, refractory hypertension. This was the removal of both adrenal glands, and replacement therapy with the life-essential hormone cortisone. The aim, said Dollery,

> was to find a precarious ledge between death from Addisonian crisis on the one hand and malignant hypertension on the other. It was a challenging experience for a preregistration house officer. If the blood pressure was brought under control there was dramatic clinical improvement. Pulmonary oedema vanished like magic, deterioration of renal function halted, and retinal cotton wool spots and papilloedema quickly regressed.

The available treatment before the development of antihypertensive drugs was reviewed by Wilkins in 1946 (5). It consisted of bed rest and reassurance of the patient, weight loss through the adoption of a low fat diet, restriction of salt intake, no smoking and possibly the use of sedatives and hypnotics to alleviate stress. As is evident, this regimen is virtually identical with that advocated by antivivisectionists today as totally effective against hypertension (1), in their attempts to dismiss the need for drug treatment and thus animal experiments. Yet malignant hypertension was then, as described above, a dreadful disease, as a last resort only treatable by the removal of a life-essential endocrine gland and consequent life-long hormone replacement (see Table below).

MALIGNANT HYPERTENSION: CASE REPORTS.
From Keith, Wagener & Kernohan (1928) *Arch Int Med* **41** 141.

Case	Sex	Age	History	BP	Duration of life from diagnosis (months)
18	F	24	Headache, visual disturbance	280/190	11
32	M	36	Headache, attacks of unconsciousness	235/135	5
38	F	15	Headache, albuminurea	200/140	11
40	F	19	Headache, dispnoea, blurred vision	270/150	1.5
46	M	28	Tachycardia, dispnoea	230/160	8
49	M	36	Constant headache	245/145	1.5

Development of Antihypertensive Therapy

The first effective treatment of severe hypertension stemmed from the study of the autonomic nervous system, that is those peripheral nerves that control the minute-by-minute activity of individual organs. Activation of the sympathetic nerves of the autonomic system was shown, in animals, to cause constriction of blood vessels and hence a rise in blood pressure. Attention was thus directed at abolishing the activity of the sympathetic nervous system in hypertension, initially by its removal or "sympathectomy." This was not an operation to be lightly undertaken and its efficacy in hypertension was never definitively established.

Of great import was the demonstration, after many experiments on various mammals, that nerves affected the organs they innervate by the release of small amounts of a chemical as each impulse reached the nerve ending. This "chemical transmission" at nerve endings provided a potential site for the use of drugs to modify nerve activity. This could be achieved either by using a synthetic chemical to mimic the effect of the "transmitter," or by the use of a chemical that could block either the release or the action of the transmitter.

Ganglionic Blocking Drugs

In all autonomic nerves there are neuron to neuron junctions (or synapses). The transmission across the synapse is achieved by the release of acetylcholine from the first neuron, which acts on a receptor on the second neuron to cause activation. The swelling in autonomic nerves which signifies where most of the synapses are present, is called a ganglion. Some quaternary ammonium compounds were shown to cause a blockade of the acetylcholine receptors at ganglia and hence a fall in blood pressure in animal experiments. This effect was however, too short-lived for clinical exploitation.

The major breakthrough in the control of severe hypertension emerged from a study of the actions of the polymethylene-bisquaternary ammonium salts in the anaesthetised cat by Paton and Zaimis in 1948 (6). These compounds consisted of two quaternised nitrogen atoms separated by a methylene chain of from 2 to 12 carbon atoms in length.

Chemical similarity with other drugs suggested that the 9-11 methylene compounds might be potent voluntary muscle relaxants, drugs of considerable importance for the control of convulsions and for use during surgery. The 10 methylene compound (decamethonium) was indeed a potent neuromuscular blocking drug. This activity decreased with shortening of the chain and was absent in the 7 methylene compound.

Fortunately, Paton and Zaimis continued with the investigation of the smaller molecules and found that they had other activity. The 5 and 6 methylene compounds markedly lowered the blood pressure of the anaesthetised cat, and on injection to the rabbit, caused the ears to flush bright red. The latter action impressed Paton, since he recalled Claude Bernard's observation almost a hundred years earlier, that cutting the sympathetic nerve to the rabbit's ear produced the same effect. Paton therefore suspected that these drugs were blocking sympathetic ganglia. Further experimentation established that this was indeed the action of the 5 and 6 methylene compounds, and Paton and Zaimis considered that the 6 methylene compound (hexamethonium) might be usable in hypertension as a "clean, specific ganglion-blocker."

It is an interesting historical aside that Paton and Zaimis originally intended to restrict their first publication on the activity of these methonium compounds to their neuromuscular blocking actions. The reason for their decision to include a mention of the possible use of hexamethonium in high blood pressure, was that the head technician of the engineering workshop in their Hampstead laboratory had malignant hypertension, and was becoming incapacitated by splitting headaches and deteriorating sight. Paton described the technician as "a beautiful craftsman" and "a very nice man." No doubt the publication of the blood pressure-lowering actions of hexamethonium hastened the clinical use of this drug for malignant hypertension, but unhappily it was too late for Paton's technician, who died soon after.

Clinical studies with hexamethonium began almost immediately in Dunedin, New Zealand, and in two centres in London (4). The treatment of malignant hypertension with hexamethonium showed that reducing the blood pressure

- relieved the severe headache;
- enabled the retinal damage to regress and hence improved vision;
- allowed the enlarged heart and oedema of the lung in hypertensive heart failure to return towards normal;
- allowed the patient to return to work (7).

Development of Antihypertensive Drugs

The realisation that the raised blood pressure in hypertension was not a compensation for the narrowing of the lumen of blood vessels, and that simply lowering the blood pressure dramatically improved the prognosis in hypertension, stimulated a tremendous research effort to produce other, improved hypotensive drugs. Although hexamethonium was of great significance since, as Paton said "it helped to get a foot in the door of really effective treatment of hypertension" (7), it had many undesirable side actions because of blockade of autonomic reflexes of the parasympathetic as well as the sympathetic system.

The development, after extensive animal experiments, of selective inhibitors of adrenergic neurones by pharmacologists at Burroughs Wellcome and the Ciba Company, provided a treatment without the unpleasant symptoms caused by block of parasympathetic ganglia (bethanidine and guanethidine). Further drug treatments for hypertension followed rapidly (4), with the development of reserpine (shown to cause hypotension in the cat (19)), hydralazine (hypotensive in dog and cat (20)), alpha methyldopa and the first thiazide diuretic, chlorothiazide (action established in dog, lack of toxicity in dog, rat and mouse (Figs. 16.1 and 16. 2).

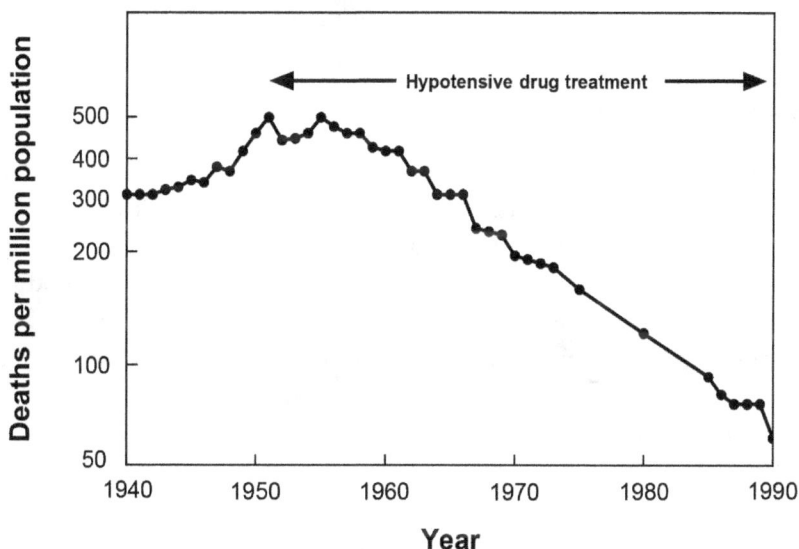

Fig. 16.1 Deaths from hypertensive disease. Annual deaths per million population. Data from Paton et al. (1978), *Highlights of British Science*, Silver Jubilee Exhibition, Royal Society and *Compendium of Health Statistics*, 8th edition, 1992 (Office of Health Economics).

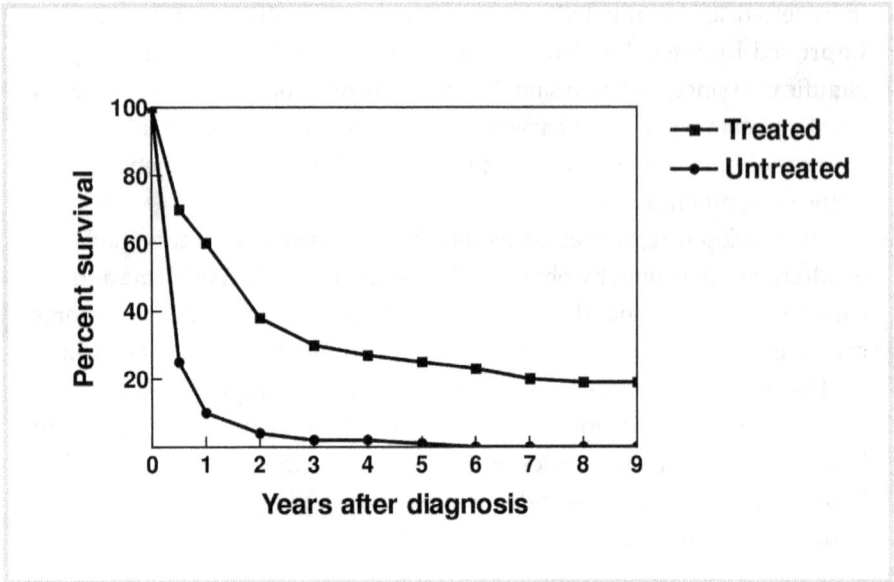

Fig. 16.2　Treatment of malignant hypertension with ganglionic blocking drugs. Comparison between 140 treated and 105 untreated patients, percent surviving against time after diagnosis. Data from Paton et al. (1978).

Beta Blockers

The use of beta blocking drugs in hypertension stemmed from the observation by Prichard that administration of pronethalol (the first beta blocker in clinical use) to patients with angina resulted in a small but persistent fall in blood pressure (8). Pronethalol was withdrawn because it was shown to produce tumours in mice, but the use of the beta blocker propranolol in hypertension was described by Prichard the same year. Comparative trials of propranolol with proven antihypertensive drugs established the value of beta blocking drugs in hypertension.

The fact that such an important antihypertensive agent emerged from clinical observation is hailed by the National Anti-Vivisection Society as an example of "progress without animals" (9). The beta blocking drugs however, were developed and perfected for the treatment of angina and some forms of cardiac arrhythmia, after years of animal experimentation. Without that animal experimental work the drugs would not have been available for clinical use. The fact that whilst being used successfully for angina an additional indication was uncovered is certainly a tribute to the acumen and persistence of the clinician, but in no way a condemnation of animal experiments.

After the hypotensive actions of propranolol were demonstrated in patients, the drug was also shown to reduce the blood pressure of spontaneously hypertensive rats (SHR) (10). These rats, as they mature, develop a high blood pressure, with consequent pathological changes in the kidneys, and cardiovascular and cerebrovascular complications similar to those that occur in patients (11). Had propranolol been tested before in SH rats, its antihypertensive activity would have been exposed. However, from all the clinical and experimental knowledge of the time, no-one could have predicted such an action. Even today, the mechanism of action of beta blockers in hypertension is not absolutely certain.

ACE Inhibitors

The discovery of the effectiveness of angiotensin converting enzyme (ACE) inhibitors in hypertension is a particularly interesting example of how animal experiments can contribute, sometimes in a circuitous way, to the development of new medicines.

Study of the effects of the venom of a Brazilian snake, *Bothrops jararaca*, led to the discovery of bradykinin, a peptide with potent pharmacological actions that could be formed in blood. The Brazilian pharmacologist Sergio Ferreira, also found in the venom a factor that markedly potentiated the actions of bradykinin. He called this bradykinin potentiating factor or BPF. In the 1960s, Ferreira brought a sample of BPF to the Royal College of Surgeons in London, where he was to work with Professor John Vane as a postdoctoral fellow. Vane's interest at this time was the biological importance of another peptide that could be formed in the blood, angiotensin II. This substance caused a marked rise in the blood pressure, and was formed from a relatively inactive precursor, angiotensin I, by a converting enzyme (ACE). It was thus inevitable that the action of BPF would eventually be tested on ACE, and it was found to be a potent inhibitor, thus preventing the production of the hypertensive angiotensin II in the body (12).

BPF was shown to reverse the rise in blood pressure produced in rats by occlusion of the renal artery, and lowered the blood pressure in other rat models of hypertension. Eventually the purified BPF was synthesised and was shown to lower the blood pressure in hypertensive patients. The preparation of a non-peptide, orally active enzyme inhibitor was thus shown to be a worthwhile therapeutic objective. The synthesis of a number of candidates, tested in rat models of hypertension, resulted in the marketing of captopril as a successful antihypertensive treatment in 1977 (12). Captopril was later also shown to be also useful in congestive heart failure.

Conclusion

The drug treatment of hypertensive disease has been a remarkable success story. From the life-saving but clumsy ganglionic blocking drugs, with their miserable side effects and poor absorption, came the graduation to improved drugs with fewer, but still severe, side actions. Often, these side actions were dose-related and thus probably preventable (4). Today the drug treatment is relatively refined. For the vast majority of patients therapy for hypertension is effective and benign. With the prospect of the development of novel drugs, such as angiotensin receptor antagonists, even further refinement might be envisaged (13). The realisation of the crucial importance of the vascular endothelial cell in the control of the calibre of vessels through the continuous release of nitric oxide (NO) (14), and the demonstration that patients with untreated hypertension possess an abnormality of the NO-mediated dilatation of arterioles (15), will no doubt furnish additional treatments or even a cure for hypertension.

Although the most striking achievement has been the control of malignant hypertension, over the last 40 years a number of clinical trials have shown that treating less extreme cases of raised blood pressure can reduce the risk of stroke, coronary heart disease and renal disease (16). Since the drug treatment of the disease has improved so much, there is a risk that it might be instituted in patients with only slightly raised diastolic pressure. Provided their blood pressure is constantly monitored, such patients might be better helped by the more conservative measures of diet, reduced salt intake etc. that were the norm prior to the 1950s. A number of thoughtful papers have recently appeared which suggest such conservative treatments might be preferable (and cheaper) than drug therapy except in high risk groups, for example those with a family history of hypertension (17). Such papers are used by antivivisectionists to claim that patients are treated unnecessarily with drugs (18). Whereas one must be vigilant to ensure that drugs are not used without sound reason, it is a clinical decision at what systolic and diastolic pressure one institutes drug therapy, and nothing to do with animal experimentation. It is indisputable that animal experiments, through providing effective hypotensive drugs, have reduced mortality and morbidity from cardiovascular and cerebrovascular disease.

An earlier version of this chapter was published as: The control of malignant hypertension. *RDS News* October 1994 6-9.

References

1) Sharpe R (1988) *The Cruel Deception: The Use of Animals in Medical Research.* London: Thorsons.

2) Schottstaedt M & Sokolow M (1953) The natural history and course of hypertension with papilledema (malignant hypertension). *Am Heart J* **45** 331.

3) Paton W (1993) Personal communication.

4) Dollery C (1987) Hypertension. *Br Heart J* **58** 179.

5) Wilkins R (1946) Essential hypertension; present status of the problem. *Med Clin N Am* **5** 1079.

6) Paton W & Zaimis E (1948) Clinical potentialities of certain bisquaternary salts causing neuromuscular and ganglionic block. *Nature* **162** 810.

7) Paton W (1982) Hexamethonium. *Br J clin Pharmac* **13** 7.

8) Prichard B (1982) Propranolol and ß-adrenergic receptor blocking drugs in the treatment of hypertension. *Br J clin Pharmac* **13** 51.

9) NAVS Leaflet (1993) Animal Experiments, the Facts.

10) Garvey H & Ram N (1975) Comparative antihypertensive effects and tissue distribution of *ßeta* adrenergic blocking drugs. *J Pharm Exper Ther* **194** 220.

11) Tobian L (1974) *Hospital Practice.* February 99.

12) Vane J (1992) The technique of cascade superfusion, in *Animal Experimentation and the Future of Medical Research* ed J Botting. London: Portland Press.

13) Brown M (1993) Angiotensin receptor blockers in essential hypertension. *The Lancet* **342** 1374.

14) Rees D, Palmer R & Moncada S (1989) Role of endothelium-derived nitric oxide in the regulation of blood pressure. *Proc Natl Acad Sci USA* **86** 3375.

15) Calver A, Collier J, Moncada S & Vallance P (1992) Effect of local intra-arterial NG-monomethyl-L-arginine in patients with hypertension: the nitric oxide dilator mechanism appears normal. *J Hypertens* **10** 1025.

16) Jackson R, Barham P, Bills J, Birch T, McLennan L, MacMahon S & Maling T (1993) Management of raised blood pressure in New Zealand: a discussion document. *BMJ* **307** 107.

17) Kawachi I & Wilson N (1990) The evolution of antihypertensive therapy. *Soc Sci Med* **31** 1239.

18) Coleman V (1994) *Betrayal of Trust.* European Medical Journal, Lynmouth

19) Sen G & Bose K (1931) *Ind Med World* **2** 194.

20) Gross F, Druey J & Meier R (1950) Eine nueu Gruppe blutdrucksenkender Substanzen von besonderem Wirkungscharakter. *Experientia* **6** 19.

21) Beyer K (1958) The mechanism of action of chlorothiazide. *Ann NY Acad Sci* **71** 363.

Acknowledgement: The late Sir William Paton was approached early in 1993 to consider writing an article on the development of the drug treatment of hypertension. He regretfully declined but was very generous with the supply of reprints and with his reminiscences of his own research and of the life of the hypertensive patient before the 1950s.

17. Penicillin And Laboratory Animals: The Animal Rights Myth

The dramatic impact of penicillin on the treatment of patients with severe infections has rightfully been paraded by biomedical researchers as a vindication of the value of laboratory animals in research. Opponents of animal experimentation are equally emphatic that animal experiments not only played no part in the development of penicillin but also that reliance on such techniques might well have caused penicillin to be discarded (1,2). The basis of the animal rights argument is that Fleming did not use animals but the "humble culture dish" (1) and that penicillin would never have been used in patients if physicians had known of its supposed inordinate and unique toxicity to guinea pigs (2). Both of these claims are incorrect and based on a superficial assessment of the literature. Fleming, after his chance observation that contamination with spores of a strain of *Penicillium* inhibited the growth of a culture of *Staphylococcus aureus*, tested the toxicity of the mould culture on animals. He reported (3):

> the toxicity to animals of powerfully antibacterial mould broth filtrate appears to be very low. Twenty c.c. injected intravenously into a rabbit were not more toxic than the same quantity of broth. Half a c.c. injected intraperitoneally to a mouse weighing about 20gm. induced no toxic symptoms.

Rather than animal experiments making no contribution to the recognition of the remarkable potential of penicillin, it has been argued that the development of this drug was in fact initially retarded by the omission of a simple and well-established animal test. The mouse protection test, whereby mice are injected intraperitoneally with pathogenic bacteria, and potential antibacterial substances administered to assess their ability to prevent death, had been described in 1911. From 1927 onwards Domagk and his team at Elberfeld

http://dx.doi.org/10.11647/OBP.0055.17

used this *in vivo* technique routinely to assess the antibacterial efficacy of the azo dyes, this work culminating in the introduction of prontosil (which was inactive *in vitro*) and hence the sulphonamides (4). Had Fleming used this test during the studies that were the basis of his 1929 paper (3) he would have found, as did Florey and his colleagues at Oxford ten years later, that his crude broth contained sufficient active substance to protect mice artificially infected with susceptible organisms.

Penicillin and the Guinea Pig

The fact that penicillin, whilst being relatively innocuous for most species, appeared to be toxic to guinea pigs and hamsters, has served as a sheet anchor for the claims of antivivisectionists that species differences render animal experiments redundant and possibly dangerous. However, the apparent sensitivity of these species to penicillin, and indeed other antibiotics, is certainly not evidence of the futility of animal experimentation It is in fact a good example of the usefulness of the appropriate model in biomedical research.

The story began with the comprehensive and careful piece of work by Dorothy Hamre and her colleagues (5). These workers were interested in the effect of penicillin on gas gangrene. They therefore administered penicillin to guinea pigs that had been infected with *Clostridium perfringens*. The animals died 12-72 hours after receiving daily doses of penicillin for 3-4 days, yet showed no signs of gas gangrene.

Hamre therefore investigated the actual toxicity of penicillin to guinea pigs and found this species, unlike mice and rabbits, to be susceptible to repeated daily doses of the antibiotic. The samples of penicillin available at this time were very impure. It is clear from Hamre's results with purer preparations that some of penicillin's immediate and delayed effects were due to impurities. Nevertheless, daily doses 7-12 times those used in patients could result in lethargy, weight loss and often (but not invariably) death after 3-7 days. However, a dose approximate to that used clinically administered even for twenty days did not kill the guinea pigs.

Hamre thus stated:

> The fact that present preparations are toxic for guinea pigs when given subcutaneously does not mean that penicillin is toxic for man. When treated with the same dose of penicillin per kg. as that given to man, guinea pigs did not die and, in fact, failed to show any signs of toxicity. *However, it is suggested that chronic toxicity for man be borne in mind* [my emphasis].

Hamre's paper was carefully written and, as subsequent research showed, to some extent prophetic.

There were occasional attempts to explain the apparent toxic effects of penicillin over the following decade, but no progress was made until a group of Belgian workers suggested that a change in the composition of the bacteria in the gut was responsible. De Somer and his colleagues showed that the Gram-positive microorganisms that inhabit guinea pig intestine are completely removed by the penicillin and are replaced by insensitive bacteria. Injection into normal guinea pigs of a sterile filtrate of a culture of these bacteria produced a condition identical to penicillin poisoning (6). It was thus supposed these new bacteria colonising the gut produced toxins that are absorbed by the guinea pigs causing the illness and perhaps death of the animals. The theory that the guinea pigs thus die from an enterocolitis, rather than from a direct toxic effect of the penicillin was supported by the observation that penicillin is not toxic to germ-free guinea pigs (7). Such animals were unaffected by penicillin 240 mg/kg/day but conventionally reared guinea pigs given this dose died within 7 days of severe infection of the colon (Fig. 17.1).

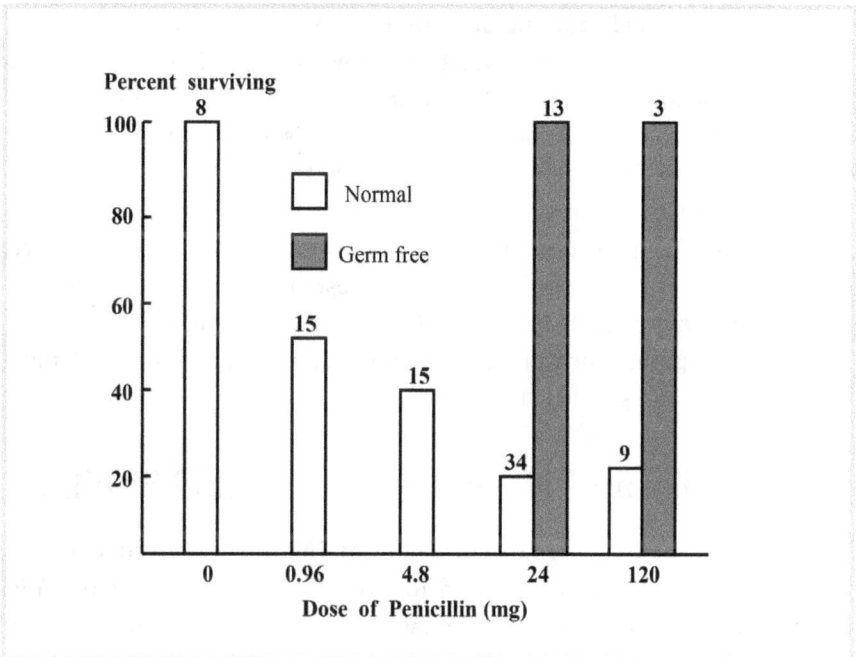

Fig. 17.1 Effect of penicillin in normal and germ-free guinea pigs. Figures are number of animals per group. Data from S. B. Formal, G. D. Abrams, H. Schneider, and R. Laundy (1963), 'Penicillin in germ-free guinea pigs.' *Nature*, 198:712.

The fact that penicillin itself is therefore not toxic is unlikely to impress the implacable opponent of animal experimentation, who requires only a simple quote for argument. However, this reaction, noted in the guinea pig in 1943, was in fact a prediction of what became, within ten years, a common iatrogenic condition in patients.

Antibiotic Associated Colitis

Pseudomembranous enterocolitis was first described in 1893 (8). It was commonly observed in post-operative patients. The characteristic of the condition is the appearance of a pseudomembrane over the gut mucosa. Microscopically the membrane can be seen to be composed of mucin, fibrin, white blood cells and sloughed mucosal epithelial cells. Occasionally the complete membrane is sloughed off and passed out as a "cast of the colon" (8).

Although most early cases of pseudomembranous colitis occurred post-operatively, antibiotics also became implicated as causative factors soon after their introduction in the 1940s (9). The location of the lesion following antibiotic use was invariably the colon rather than the small intestine, thus this particular condition was named "antimicrobial-induced pseudomembranous colitis."

The cause of the condition was the removal of sensitive bacteria from the gut by the antibiotic. This then results in profound alterations in the composition of the gut microflora due to recolonisation of the gut by other micro-organisms. This phenomenon was noted to follow administration of penicillin given by mouth or by injection. Generally the change in intestinal flora produced by penicillin (and other antibiotics) was of no significance, since the normal intestinal flora became re-established after therapy was stopped. In some patients however, after prolonged administration of the antibiotic, a superinfection occurred in the gut resulting in life-threatening pseudomembranous colitis (10).

Guinea Pigs and Humans: Remarkably Similar

The particular micro-organism recolonising the gut and causing pseudomembranous colitis eluded identification for many years. This, sometimes fatal, condition was originally attributed to mucosal ischaemia or a viral infection. Ultimately stools from affected patients were shown to contain a toxin that damaged cultured cells (11). Shortly after, this toxin was shown to be derived from *Clostridium difficile* (12, 13). It thus appeared that *C.*

difficile was the pathogen that caused pseudomembranous colitis. This was not easy for everyone to accept. *C. difficile* had been described in 1935 (14). It was difficult to isolate and slow to grow in culture (thus it was designated the "difficult clostridium"). As it was found in the stools of quite healthy infants *C. difficile* was considered to be innocuous and thus of little interest. When it became clear that infants are resistant to the effects of *C. difficile* toxin only until about 12 months of age (possibly due to the absence of toxin receptors on the immature cells of their gut (11) it became generally accepted that *C. difficile* was a pathogen and indeed the cause of pseudomembranous colitis.

Returning to the animal studies, veterinary research has strengthened the apparent similarity between guinea pigs and humans. Penicillin-induced inflammation of the large intestine of guinea pigs has been shown to be caused by clostridial toxins, and *C. difficile* has been isolated from the gut contents of these animals (16). Newborn guinea pigs, like germ-free animals, have been shown *not* to be susceptible to penicillin (17). Perhaps neonatal guinea pigs, like babies under 12 months of age, are insensitive to clostridial toxins.

It is clear that the now common, clinical problem of antibiotic-induced colitis (15) is analogous to the condition observed in guinea pigs by Hamre and her colleagues 50 years ago. An intensive investigation of the effects of penicillin on the intestinal flora of the guinea pig might have forewarned clinicians of the life-threatening superinfections that can occur with prolonged use of some antimicrobials. However it would be uncharitable to suggest the early experimental workers in the field were remiss. On the contrary, the admonition by Hamre that "chronic toxicity (of penicillin) for man be borne in mind" was an accurate and perceptive observation.

There is no basis for citing the effect of penicillin on guinea pigs as a prime example of species difference; in fact, it is an example of the exact opposite, namely of strikingly similar effects on the guinea pig and on people. The misrepresentation of the history of penicillin is but one example of the distortion of scientific fact perpetrated by opponents of animal research. It is the responsibility of scientists to correct these errors before they gain unwarranted credibility with the general public.

An earlier version of this chapter was published as: Burying the penicillin myth. *RDS News* July 1995 6-7.

References

1) Sharpe R (1988) *The Cruel Deception: The Use of Animals in Medical Research.* London: Thorsons.

2) Ruesch, H (1982) *Naked Empress.* Klosters: Civis Publications.

3) Fleming, A (1929) On the antibacterial action of cultures of a Penicillium, with special reference to their use in the isolation of B. influenzae. *Br. J. Exp. Pathol,* **10** 226-36.

4) Florey, H (1953) The advance of chemotherapy by animal experiment. *Conquest* **41** 4-14.

5) Hamre, D M, Rake, G, McKee, C M and MacPhillamy, H B (1943) The toxicity of penicillin as prepared for clinical use. *Am. J. Med. Sci.* **206** 642-52.

6) De Somer, P, Van De Voorde, H, Eyssen, H and Van Dijck, P (1955) A study on penicillin toxicity in guinea pigs. *Ant. Chemother* **5** 463-69.

7) Formal, S B, Abrams, G D Schneider, H and Laundy, R (1963) Penicillin in germ-free guinea pigs. *Nature* **198** 712.

8) Finney, J M T (1893) Gastroenterostomy for cicatrizing ulcer of the pylorus. *Bull. Johns. Hopkins Hosp.* **4** 53.

9) Bartlett, J G and Gorbach, S L (1977) Pseudomembranous enterocolitis (antibiotic-related colitis). *Adv. Int. Med.* **22** 455-76.

10) Mandell, G L and Sande, M A (1990) Penicillins, cephalosporins and other beta-lactam antibiotics, in Gilman, A G, Rall, T W, Nies, A S. and Taylor, P. eds. *Goodman & Gilman's The Pharmacological Basis of Therapeutics.* 8th edition. New York: Pergamon Press, pp. 1065-97.

11) Kelly, C P, Pothoulakis, C. and LaMont, J T (1994) *Clostridium difficile* colitis. *New Eng. J. Med.* **330** 257-62.

12) Bartlett, J G, Chang, T W, Gurwith, M, Gorbach, S L and Onderdonk, A B (1978) Antibiotic-associated pseudomembranous colitis due to toxin-producing clostridia. *New. Eng. J. Med.* **298** 531-34.

13) Larson, H E, Price, A B, Honour, P and Borriello, S P (1978) *Clostridium difficile* and the aetiology of pseudomembranous colitis. *The Lancet* **1** 1063-66.

14) Hall, I C and O'Toole, E (1935) Intestinal flora in new-born infants with a description of a new pathogenic anaerobe. *Bacillus difficilis. Am. J. Dis. Child.* **49** 390-402.

15) Anon. (1995) Antibiotic-induced diarrhoea. *DTB* **33** 23-24.

16) Lowe, B R, Fox, J G and Bartlett, J G (1980) *Clostridium difficile*-associated cecitis in guinea pigs exposed to penicillin. *Am. J. Vet. Res.* **41** 1277-1279.

17) Manning, P J Wagner, J F and Harkness, J E (1984) Biology and diseases of guinea pigs, in Fox, J, Cohen, B and Loew, F eds. *Laboratory Animal Medicine.* New York: Academic Press, p. 173.

18. The History of Thalidomide

No drug has had a greater effect than thalidomide on the extent and intensity of the preclinical investigation of potential medicines required by the regulatory authorities. Indeed, the establishment of thalidomide as the cause of the apparent epidemic of children born with horrific deformities in the late 1950s was responsible for the institution of some regulatory bodies, such as the United Kingdom's Committee on the Safety of Drugs, and for the strengthening of others, such as the Food and Drugs Administration (FDA) of the United States. Despite this, the history of the development of thalidomide, and of the subsequent studies of the teratogenic and other effects of the drug, has become confused, because of misrepresentation by those anxious to discredit the contribution of animal experimentation to medical advances.

Two categorical statements can be made about thalidomide. First, thalidomide was never administered to pregnant animals before it was used in humans. Secondly, only five months after the teratogenic effects of thalidomide had been established and the drug withdrawn, embryopathic actions of thalidomide were shown to occur in rat and rabbit (1). Over the following ten years fetal malformations caused by thalidomide were demonstrated in seven other species of small mammal and eight species of monkey (2).

Early Experimental Studies

The first paper describing the pharmacological actions of thalidomide was published in 1956 by Kunz, Keller and Mückter from the Research Laboratories of the German pharmaceutical firm Chemie Grünenthal (3). Thalidomide, designated then as K17, was alleged to reduce spontaneous movement in mice without the initial excitement phase observed with other sedative drugs

http://dx.doi.org/10.11647/OBP.0055.18

such as phenobarbitone and glutethimide. The onset of action of thalidomide was rapid and the sedative effect more profound and of longer duration of action than that of the comparator drugs. Coordination, as detected by ability of mice to cling to a slowly rotating rod, was not reduced even with doses in excess of those that produced sedation. Of greater significance, thalidomide was claimed to be virtually non-toxic, oral doses in excess of 5000mg/kg failing to cause death, whereas 600mg/kg and 300mg/kg doses of glutethimide and phenobarbitone respectively were sufficient to kill half of the mice in a test group. Chronic administration of 100-500mg/kg thalidomide to mice, rats, guinea pigs and rabbits for 30 days appeared to be well-tolerated. Thus it was proposed by the researchers at Chemie Grünenthal that thalidomide would be a useful sedative or hypnotic that did not carry the suicide risk of contemporary medicines.

Of significance, the authors emphasised that thalidomide was poorly water soluble but claimed, with no evidence, that the apparent innocuity is "not only due to the fact that the compound is sparingly soluble in water; it also indicates extremely low toxicity." Crucially, no measurements of blood or tissue concentrations of thalidomide in treated animals were performed. Such data would have demonstrated that the lack of toxicity of thalidomide was indeed due to lack of absorption of the drug. The paper by Kunz, Keller and Mückter that appeared in *Arzneimittel-Forschung* was immediately followed by a clinical report by Jung (4) describing the sedative effects of thalidomide in 300 patients who were given 25-200 mg thalidomide three times a day. There was no comparison with a placebo group and no indication of the duration of treatment was given. The blood picture of 20 of the patients was alleged to be unchanged over 4 weeks and liver function tests in 20 patients with enlarged livers showed no abnormality. However, no numerical data was provided to support these claims. With high doses side effects included sleepiness, giddiness and constipation. Some thirty years after the publication of these papers, the pediatrician Widukind Lenz, who played a significant part in the exposure of thalidomide as the cause of embryopathy, stated: "The papers published in 1956 by Kunz et al. on animal experiments and by Jung on clinical experiences with thalidomide have so little scientific value that in my opinion they should not have been accepted for print." (5)

The actions of thalidomide were also investigated by G. B. Somers (6), chief pharmacologist at the Distillers Company, which was licensed by Grünenthal to distribute thalidomide in the British and Commonwealth markets. Somers, using thalidomide as a suspension in 1% carboxymethylcellulose, generally confirmed the inhibition of spontaneous movement by the drug in mice and also remarked on its apparent lack of toxicity in animals. However, Somers added an important caveat when discussing the results of his toxicity studies: "It may well be that the absence of toxicity is due to a limited absorption, for the compound has a low solubility in body fluids, and when administered parenterally remains at the site of injection. In the absence of a suitable assay method absorption studies have not yet been made."

Somers was later proved correct. Some months after his initial experiments he tested the actions of thalidomide prepared as a finely ground suspension in sugar solution. Such a preparation had just been marketed by Grünenthal as a sedative *Contergan Saft* that allegedly could be safely used by children. Somers was shocked to discover that microfined thalidomide mixed with sugar solution, unlike the suspensions originally used, was highly toxic to mice (7).

Even by the standards of the time, the preclinical and clinical investigation of thalidomide was superficial. This is illustrated by the animal studies performed upon meprobamate, a muscle relaxant and sedative agent first described by Berger in 1954 (8). Acute toxicity was measured in rats after oral administration and intraperitoneal injection, and in mice via these routes as well as after intravenous injection. Acute toxicity was also measured in monkeys. Subacute toxicity was examined in dogs given 1 g of meprobamate daily for between 60-75 days. The blood picture, urine analysis and kidney function tests were performed before administration of the drug and 30 and 60 days after treatment; blood urea nitrogen and urea clearance were measured at 60 days. At autopsy, dogs showed no abnormalities of kidney, stomach, small intestine, liver, bladder or adrenal glands. Chronic toxicity studies were performed over 15 months on five groups of 20 male and female rats. Two groups were used as controls, the remaining groups received 2%, 1% or 0.5% meprobamate in the diet. At the 12th week, male and female animals were mated and the resulting neonates examined for normality. There were no differences between control and test groups in the intensive examinations of the blood and urine, and the histological examination of all the major organs at autopsy. Unlike the relatively superficial preclinical examination of thalidomide reported two years later, Berger looked at the fate of meprobamate in the body, examining the urine for breakdown products. Approximately 10% of the drug was excreted unchanged in the urine, a much greater percentage excreted in a conjugated form, partly as an unknown metabolite conjugated with glucuronide.

Clinical Usage

On the basis of the limited experimental studies, and further clinical trials (none double blind), thalidomide was launched in Germany in November, 1957 as a novel "non-toxic" sedative under the trade name *Contergan*, although it had had limited use as a component, together with quinine, phenacetin, salicylate and vitamin C, of an anti-influenza preparation termed *Grippex* since November 1956 (9).

Contergan was marketed aggresively as a completely harmless sedative, and as a result its sales increased markedly throughout 1959. However, its alleged lack of toxicity soon came into question. In October 1959 a neurologist, Dr R Voss diagnosed polyneuritis in three patients who had taken *Contergan* for a year, and raised with Grünenthal his concern that the drug might have a toxic action on peripheral nerves. Despite the fact that, from April 1959, Grünenthal representatives had received information from pharmacists and physicians that *Contergan* caused numerous side effects including abnormally cold hands and feet, paraesthesia and giddiness, Grünenthal replied to Voss saying "no such side effects have come to our notice" (10).

Nonetheless Voss described his three cases at a neurological congress in Düsseldorf on April 30th 1960. The presentation by Voss prompted numerous other reports of apparent severe peripheral neuritis in long-term users of *Contergan*. Frenkel, a neurologist from Königstein, who like Voss had contacted Grünenthal earlier with concerns about the safety of *Contergan*, submitted a paper to *Medizinische Welt* describing 20 patients he believed to have thalidomide-induced peripheral neuritis. Grünenthal representatives attempted to persuade Frenkel to withdraw or delay publication but he refused. However, for reasons that are unclear, Frenkel's paper did not appear in print until May 6th, 1961. This was well after the first literature report describing thalidomide-induced peripheral neuritis which was from Dr A. Leslie Florence of Aberdeenshire, United Kingdom. In a letter to the *British Medical Journal* of December 31st 1960, entitled "Is thalidomide to blame," Florence described 4 patients presenting with marked paraesthesia affecting first the feet then the hands, coldness of the extremities, ataxia and nocturnal cramp. All patients had been taking thalidomide for between eighteen months to two years. Cessation of the drug resulted in alleviation but not removal of the symptoms (11). By the end of May 1961 there were at least 1,300 cases of peripheral neuritis associated with long-term thalidomide therapy, and Grünenthal were forced to take steps to have the drug supplied only on prescription. This side action was soon to appear to be insignificant compared to the catastrophic result of ingestion of the drug by women during days 35-50 of their pregnancy, but the broad dissemination of the fact that thalidomide caused nerve damage was partially responsible for alerting Frances Kelsey, the FDA medical officer responsible for evaluating thalidomide before its use in the USA, to the fact that this supposed non-toxic medicine was potentially dangerous. The consequent delay in the approval of thalidomide until after its teratogenic effects were established in Europe thus averted a disaster for the United States (12).

Thalidomide and Fetal Abnormalities

The first indication of the emergence in Germany of an epidemic of particular fetal deformities was the description in 1959 by a Munich gynaecologist, Weidenbach, of a child with phocomelia of the arms and legs (13). Weidenbach knew this to be a highly unusual type of deformity since he could find no silmilar case in the German literature, nor had any case been described in the records of the Bavarian Institution for Crippled Children since its institution in 1913 (six years later, in 1965, four years after thalidomide had been withdrawn in Germany, Weidenbach finally established that the mother of the deformed child had been prescribed the thalidomide-containing preparation *Grippex* for a febrile condition between the 25th and 35th day post conception).

Other sporadic cases were reported but strong evidence that these fetal abnormalities had a common exogenous cause only emerged in September 1960, when Kosenow and Pfeiffer, at a meeting of the German Paediatric Association, presented details of two cases of children born with severe skeletal malformations together with various other deformities such as duodenal stenosis and capillary hemangioma of the upper lip. Of great significance, both children had been born on consecutive days (February 28th and 29th) in the same small German town. Some years later it was finally established that both mothers had been prescribed thalidomide between the 44th and 46th postmenstrual day (9).

By the beginning of 1961 it was clear that there was an epidemic of limb deformities in Germany, typically shortening or absence of the long bones of the arms or legs, producing flipper- or seal-like limbs, the condition designated "phocomelia." Lenz was certain that one single common cause was responsible (14). He asked one affected parent specifically whether any new drugs had been taken during pregnancy. He received a detailed list of the diet and diseases of the mother and a list of ten drugs. *Contergan* was not mentioned.

By August 1961, Lenz estimated that the incidence of gross defects of the long bones had increased 10-fold in Hamburg and probably 100-fold or more in some towns of Rhineland and Westphalia. In September, 1961 Wiedeman published a paper in which he described seeing in his clinic in Krefeld only four cases of limb deformity between 1950-59, but 13 cases in the last 10 months (14). Careful investigation excluded infection, irradiation, anticonception chemicals and attempted abortion as possible causes, but Wiedeman was convinced that a newly introduced toxic factor was responsible.

Thalidomide (as *Contergan*) was originally considered as a candidate by the paediatrician Weicker, who in August 1961 had collected detailed data on 20 cases, and found *Contergan* was mentioned in five. Unfortunately, he ignored the possible connection since he was mistakenly informed that thalidomide was widely used in the United States, where no cases of phocomelia had occurred (12). In November 1961 Lenz visited two further cases and established that both mothers had taken *Contergan* during pregnancy. Lenz told Weicker of his suspicions and the latter rechecked his now considerable collection of case histories and found 34 cases with positive evidence of thalidomide use by the mother. Encouraged by this and other confirmatory evidence from Professors Wiedeman (Kiel) and Kosenow (Krefeld), Lenz telephoned Grünenthal describing his concern. He was told he would be visited by representatives of the firm within a few days. Lenz considered the problem too serious for delay and, on November 16th, 1961 sent to Grünenthal a registered express letter detailing his reasons for assuming a connection between use of *Contergan* in early pregnancy and consequent birth defects, particularly limb deformities (14).

In Australia, where thalidomide was marketed as *Distaval* by the Distillers Company, the connection between the drug and fetal abnormalities was deduced rather more rapidly through the perception of the obstetrician McBride. On May 4, 1961 at the Women's Hospital, Sydney, McBride delivered a baby with bowel atresia and phocomelia of both arms. An obstetrician of 7 years standing, this was the first case of phocomelia McBride had seen at this hospital where there were 4,000 births each year. Twenty days later another child with similar limb malformations was delivered at the hospital. Two cases could be a coincidence, but when a third case with similar limb malformations was delivered on June 8th, 1961 McBride's suspicions were acutely aroused. Over the following days he examined the literature on drug-induced malformations and consequently examined the case notes dealing with the three pregnancies; the only drug administered to the mothers was *Distaval*.

On June 13th, 1961 McBride persuaded the Medical Superintendent at the Women's Hospital to withdraw thalidomide from use. McBride also attempted to initiate some animal experiments, firstly using mice and guinea pigs kept at the hospital for diagnostic purposes. Lack of sufficient animals and McBride's understandable lack of expertise prompted him to approach, on two occasions, the professor of pharmacology at the University of Sydney to suggest he examine the possible teratogenic potential of thalidomide in laboratory animals. Unfortunately, the professor was not convinced by McBride's circumstantial evidence and did not consider the expense of an animal study justified (15).

McBride informed representatives of Distillers in Australia of his suspicions that thalidomide might be responsible for producing fetal abnormalities, and was assured by them that his anxieties would be transmitted to the London office. McBride nonetheless drafted a letter to the prestigious medical journal *The Lancet* stating that although congenital abnormalities can be expected in approximately 1.5% of babies, he had observed that the incidence of multiple severe abnormalities in babies delivered of women who were given the drug thalidomide during pregnancy to be almost 20%. McBride's letter, which appeared on December 16, 1961 was the first published record of the possible teratogenic action of thalidomide (16).

Distillers received the report of McBride's concern from their Australian representatives on November 21, 1961. This, together with the co-incidental information from Lenz in Germany resulted in the withdrawal of thalidomide from the German and British markets. The incidence of thalidomide-induced deformity in Germany, together with a record of other significant observations is depicted in Figure 1.

With 50 years hindsight, some may view with incredulity the delay in the association of thalidomide with the ever increasing number of cases of severe congenital defects. Yet even in April 1962, Josef Warkany, then probably the most distinguished expert on teratogenic agents, expressed doubts that thalidomide was the cause of the epidemic of limb defects, since some mothers who had taken thalidomide during pregnancy produced normal offspring, and some mothers who gave birth to children with phocomelia claimed not to have taken the drug (17). These doubts disappeared when it was established that mothers who took thalidomide after the sensitive period of 50 days into pregnancy could have normal children; and mothers who did not believe they had taken the drug could have taken it unknowingly, since it was present in some preparations without being specifically named (18). As Warkany stated: "The real proof came when disappearance of the epidemic followed withdrawal of the drug from the market." (18) (See Figure 18.1)

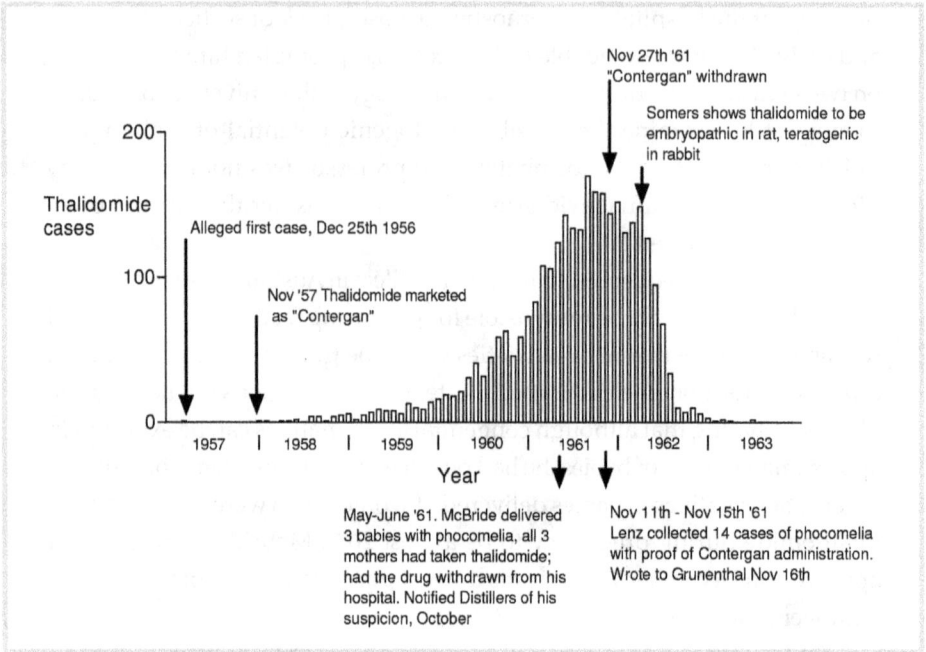

Fig. 18.1 Columns represent the monthly incidence in Germany of births of children deformed because of ingestion of thalidomide by the mother. Data was collected by the meticulous retrospective epidemiological studies of Widukind Lenz (5). The first case occurred in December, 1956. The child's father worked for Chemie Grünenthal and had received samples of thalidomide tablets for his wife. The association of the abnormalities with administration of thalidomide was not suspected until May 1961 in Australia, and November 1961 in Germany. The rapid fall in incidence of deformity after withdrawal of thalidomide confirmed that thalidomide was responsible. In April 1962, 5 months after the withdrawal of the drug, Somers was the first to demonstrate the embryopathic action of thalidomide in animals.

Experimental Studies

Upon hearing of the concerns of Lenz and McBride, the chief pharmacologist of Distillers in Britain, Dr George Somers, launched studies of the effect of thalidomide on the fetus. Thus November 1961, after the withdrawal of the drug, was the first time thalidomide was administered to pregnant animals, apart from the unsophisticated attempts by McBride four months previously.

Somers published his results barely five months later, on 28 April 1962 also in a letter to *The Lancet* (1). In this letter he stated that thalidomide given to pregnant rabbits resulted in the birth of neonates in which: "The front legs were foreshortened owing to a reduction in long-bone formation of the radius and ulna; while the rear legs showed a varus deformity involving the tibiofibula."

Therefore, within six months of the suggested association between thalidomide and human fetal deformity, it had been possible to produce in a common laboratory animal a teratogenic effect identical to one of the many produced by thalidomide in humans. Surely this was evidence for a striking similarity between mammalian species rather than for a manifest difference. Somers used a dose (150 mg/kg) that was higher than that used in humans. Somers simply wanted to know if thalidomide was teratogenic in rabbit and thus did not carry out a dose-response study, which would have been wasteful of animal life. However, he subsequently obtained the same effects with a 30 mg/kg dose as did Seller with 50 mg/kg (19). Somers also later measured plasma concentrations of thalidomide after oral administration of suspensions in carboxymethylcellulose and found that with doses of 150 mg/kg the peak plasma concentration in rabbits was only three-times as high as those in humans on normal doses (19).

Within a further six months, again in *The Lancet*, a report appeared describing the teratogenic effects of thalidomide in the Sprague Dawley rat (20) and this was confirmed by other reports (21). However, a more common response of the rat fetus to the challenge of thalidomide was intrauterine death followed by resorption. In the two years following the withdrawal of thalidomide approximately 20 papers were published that reported decreased litter sizes, together with numerous uterine resorption sites, in rats given the drug during pregnancy. Christie (22), who also reported a significant increase in resorptions in thalidomide-treated pregnant rats, suggested that fetal abnormalities produced in the rat embryos might well be of sufficient severity to kill the embryo and thus account for the increase in resorption.

Other papers subsequently appeared showing negative effects of thalidomide on the fetuses of laboratory animals. Obviously, when such conflicting results occur one assumes that the negative results are wrong, for there may be many reasons for a false negative, but a positive result is unlikely to be due to chance provided adequate controls are carried out. There were probably a number of factors responsible for the false negative results. Teratology was an orphan discipline in the 1960s, with few practitioners. Inexperienced experimentalists were possibly not aware that laboratory animals, which generally give birth at night, cannibalise their pups if they are born deformed, thus the litters should be delivered by Cesarean section at term to be sure of detecting deformed neonates. Also, detecting deformities (particularly of the skeleton) in fetuses of small laboratory animals such as rats and mice is not easy; the technique of staining with alizarin dye is necessary. King and Kendrick (20) for example, found that they could double the detection of skeletal defects in rat by alizarin staining of the skeleton.

The most significant reason for the false negative results was exposed by the definitive biochemical studies of thalidomide by the group led by Professor R.T. Williams at St Mary's Hospital in London. Williams and his colleagues established that the distinct optical isomers of thalidomide were far more toxic than the mixture of the isomers (the racemate) (23). Subsequent studies of the relative effects of the separate enantiomers in the rat suggested that the teratogenic action was due to the S(-)-enantiomer. Since there is a rapid interconversion of the two isomers *in vivo* the role of stereochemical factors in thalidomide teratogenesis is probably significant but unresolved (24). Of greater significance, Williams et al. also showed that thalidomide was inherently unstable, rapidly breaking down to 12 inactive metabolites if in aqueous solution above pH 6 (25). It is probable that many workers were using solutions containing only the inactive metabolites of thalidomide and therefore obtained no fetal abnormalities. This is particularly likely, since in the British patent specification (1957) Grünenthal, commenting on the lack of solubility of thalidomide, stated quite erroneously, that thalidomide "is soluble in strong lyes, the solution obtained being yellowish in colour" (26). Such a treatment would result in the instantaneous breakdown of the substance. Chemical breakdown was certainly the reason for the apparent lack of teratogenic activity in rabbit reported by Fox et al. (27). Schumacher (28) repeated these experiments and showed that the procedures used by Fox to solubilise thalidomide resulted in considerable chemical breakdown, an observation subsequently accepted by Fox (29). Schumacher also emphasised the facilitating effect of carboxymethylcellulose (a suspending agent frequently used to make supersaturated solutions of thalidomide for experimental use) on hydrolysis. Carboxymethylcellulose contains from 7 to 8.5% sodium and therefore would tend to buffer the solution, maintaining the alkaline milieu that would foster the hydrolysis of thalidomide (28).

Unfortunately, many early papers on the experimental production of abnormalities in laboratory animals neglected to record how solutions or suspensions of thalidomide were prepared and for how long they were stored, but it is likely that negative results may well be explained by lack of absorption of the drug or the inadvertent administration of hydrolysis products rather than thalidomide itself. By 1967, Meredith Runner had stated that the embryos of all mammals so far studied are affected by thalidomide (30) and in 1989, Schardein and Keller listed 17 mammalian species in which thalidomide produced fetal abnormalities (2). It also produces limb deformities in the newt (31).

Thalidomide and the Regulation of Drug Use

The catastrophic effects of thalidomide on the developing fetus shook the confidence of the general public in the pharmaceutical industry. The dramatic improvement in the treament of infective diseases such as puerperal sepsis, pneumonia and streptococcal septicemia by the sulphonamides and penicillin, and the control of tuberculosis by streptomycin, isoniazid and aminosalicylic acid were all forgotten amid the realisation that there was no procedure in place that could prevent the marketing of a medicine that manifested a horrific toxic effect. As stated by the British Minister of Health, the Right Honourable Kenneth Robinson in May 1963: "The House and the public suddenly woke up to the fact that any drug manufacturer could market any product however inadequately tested, however dangerous, without having to satisfy any independent body as to its efficacy and safety and the public was almost uniquely unprotected in this respect." (32)

To remedy this situation a joint subcommittee of the English and Scottish Standing Medical Advisory Committees was set up to advise the Government on suitable measures to ensure that potential medicines were subjected to intensive preclinical investigation to establish their pharmacological and possible toxic actions, and to confirm their efficacy and safety in the clinic. A further remit of the Subcommittee was to advise on procedures to ensure early detection of untoward effects that may emerge after the marketing of the product and its widespread use in patients. After discussions with the Association of the British Pharmaceutical Industry (ABPI) and other professional bodies the Subcommittee recommended that the responsibility for the preclinical investigation of new drugs should remain with the individual manufacturer and that there should be an expert body created that would review the evidence and offer advice on the toxicity of new drugs. Thus, in June, 1963 the Committee on the Safety of Drugs was established under the chairmanship of Professor Derrick Dunlop (later to become Sir Derrick). It became the responsibility of this committee to assess the data presented in support of each preparation and to consider whether it may be released for marketing. The assessment of the experimental studies on the toxicity of the drug was the responsibility of a subcommittee on toxicity (32). As a minimum requirement this subcommittee would expect the drug to have been tested according to the recommendations in the report prepared for the ABPI by the Expert Committee on Drug Toxicity (33). This report describes in detail the recommendations for the general investigation of the acute, subacute and chronic toxicity of a compound, its possible carcinogenicity and its liability to interact in a toxic fashion with concurrent medication. Not surprisingly, since the stimulus for the institution of regulations governing the marketing of drugs was the toxic action of thalidomide on the fetus, the report recommended particular tests to examine possible effects of the drug on fetal development.

The recommendations were that two species should be used to study toxic effects upon the fetus, the mouse or rat, and the rabbit. Test groups should be large enough to ensure 5 pregnant animals in the control rodent group and 3 in the rabbit. Three doses of the test drug should be used: the maximum dose tolerated by the mother, a second dose large enough to produce clinically relevant effects, and an intermediate dose. Dosing should begin on day one of pregnancy and continue until the day before term. On the day before term the animals should be killed, the uteri should be removed and examined for number of resorption sites, and the number and weight of live, dead or abnormal fetuses should be determined. From this preliminary test a range of doses should be selected to establish the threshold dose for fetal loss or any aspect of fetal toxicity. In this main test, the number and weight of progeny should be monitored up to weaning, when the progeny are killed and examined externally and internally. The normality of the skeleton should be observed after staining with alizarin red.

There is no doubt that if these premarketing procedures, instituted in the early 1960s, had been applied to thalidomide its toxicity to the developing embryo would have been detected. Unlike the situation in the United Kingdom, the United States did have some legislation to regulate the marketing of novel medications. New drug applications had to be submitted to the Food and Drug Administration (FDA) to be cleared for marketing, which at that time was on the basis of safety claims alone. The FDA had 60 days to decide if the safety data supplied was adequate. A failure to communicate by day 60 would mean automatic approval of the drug. An American pharmaceutical company signed an agreement with Grünenthal to market thalidomide in the United States and submitted an application for approval to the FDA on September 12 1960. According to Frances Kelsey, the medical officer assigned to the review of the thalidomide application, "Deficiencies in all areas were found during the initial review and in several subsequent resubmissions" (12). Kelsey was particularly concerned about the report of peripheral neuritis as a side effect, of which the FDA were only informed in February 1961, despite the fact that in Britain thalidomide had carried a warning of the risk of peripheral neuritis since September 1960. The severity of peripheral neuritis as a side effect led to questions of its use during pregnancy, since the application had described its use for the treatment of insomnia in pregnancy; yet there were no data as to whether it was safe to use in this condition (12). The legitimate concerns raised by Kelsey delayed the approval of thalidomide until its withdrawal from the market in Europe and Australia in November, 1961.

Even though the requirements of the FDA and Kelsey's perception prevented the marketing of thalidomide in the United States, a few cases of thalidomide deformity did occur there since the company seeking approval to sell the drug distributed free samples of thalidomide tablets to over a thousand doctors who administered them to an estimated 20,000 patients. The realisation that potentially noxious medicines could be administered to patients prior to the approval by the FDA resulted in the Kefauver-Harris Amendment, which required that the FDA should monitor all stages of drug development before its use in humans (12).

Misrepresentation

An objective examination of published papers and contemporary accounts confirms that the preclinical tests upon thalidomide were cursory in the extreme, and there is no doubt that it was never administered to pregnant animals prior to its use in patients. Further, within a short time of thalidomide's withdrawal from the market due to its suspected association with fetal abnormalities, it was shown to produce fetal toxicity in laboratory animals. Clearly, the disaster occurred because of insufficient testing in laboratory animals.

Antivivisection organisations are however loath to accept that the thalidomide disaster offers no propaganda for their cause, asserting in leaflets and newspaper advertisements that "The thalidomide disaster is just one example of how vivisection damages us." (34) In the United Kingdom the Advertising Standards Authority (ASA) ensures that all advertisements should be "legal, decent, honest and truthful, and when capable of objective assessment, data should be supported by evidence." Upon assessing the above statement the ASA ruled that: "The common claim, that thalidomide was tested in various species and did not show the teratogenic effects that it had in humans, was considered unjustified." The agency therefore requested that reference to thalidomide in this context in future advertising be omitted (35).

Unfortunately, there are no strictures on the perpetration of misrepresentations in general literature. One of the more bizarre descriptions of the history of thalidomide is that of Greek and Greek, who state that some toxicity tests were carried out on pregnant rodents prior to thalidomide's release (36). This is not so. In fact one of the lines of defense used by the suppliers of the drug was that safety tests were not normally carried out on pregnant animals at the time thalidomide was developed. However, the preclinical investigation of meprobamate (described above) shows this claim to be false. Greek and Greek also state that it was known for five years that thalidomide was teratogenic in humans but "since animal testing had not indicated a problem with thalidomide, its use persisted. Hence animal testing delayed the recall of this highly teratogenic drug." The reviews by Lenz, Warkany and Kelsey, the leading protagonists in this field, published as the proceedings of a symposium to commemorate the 25th anniversary of the American Society of Teratology (5, 12, 17), show that the account by Greek and Greek is wildly inaccurate. However such propaganda has been eagerly grasped by antivivisectionists and widely quoted in letters to the press and in internet discussions. The public must be constantly reminded of the facts before they are swamped by the erroneous, emotive rhetoric of the opponents of animal experiments.

An earlier version of this chapter was published as: Botting, J. The history of thalidomide. *Drug News and Perspectives* 2002, **15**(9): 604-11. Copyright 2002-2014 Prous Science, S.A.U. or its licensors. All rights reserved, http://dx.doi.org/10.1358/dnp.2002.15.9.840066

References

1) Somers, G F (1962) Thalidomide and congenital abnormalities. *The Lancet* **1** 912.

2) Schardein, J L and Keller, K A (1989) Potential of human developmental toxicants and the role of animal testing in their identification and characterisation. *CRC Crit. Rev. Toxicol.* **19** 251-330.

3) Kunz, K, Keller, H and Mückter H (1956) N-Phthalyl-glutaminsäure-imid. *Arzneim.-Forsch.* **6** 426-30.

4) Jung, H (1956) Klinische Erfahrungen mit ein neuen Sedativen. *Arzneim.-Forsch.* **6** 430-32.

5) Lenz, W (1988) A short history of thalidomide embryopathy. *Teratology* **38** 203-15.

6) Somers, G F (1960) Pharmacological properties of thalidomide (α-phthalimido glutarimide), a new sedative hypnotic drug. *Brit. J. Pharmacol.* **15** 111-16.

7) Sunday Times of London (1979). *Suffer the Children: The Story of Thalidomide.* London: Andre Deutsch, p. 59.

8) Berger, F M (1954) The pharmacological properties of 2 methyl-2-N-propyl, 3 propanediol dicarbamate (Miltown), a new interneuronal blocking agent. *J. Pharmacol.Exp. Ther.* **112** 413-23.

9) Lenz, W (1979) Thalidomide: facts and inferences, in *Drug-Induced Sufferings. Int. Congr. Ser. No. 513. Proc. Kyoto Int Conf Against Drug-Induced Sufferings*, pp. 103-09.

10) As Ref. 7. p. 32.

11) Florence, A L (1960) Is thalidomide to blame? *Brit. Med. J.* **2** 1954.

12) Kelsey, F O (1988) Thalidomide update: regulatory aspects. *Teratology* 38221-25.

13) McBride, W G (1977) Thalidomide embryopathy. *Teratology* **16** 79-82.

14) Lenz, W (1985) Thalidomide Embryopathy in Germany, 1959-1961. *Prevention of Physical and Mental Congenital Defects, Part C: Basic and Medical Science, Education, and Future Strategies*, pp. 77-83.

15) As Ref. 7. pp. 86-95.

16) McBride, W G (1961) Thalidomide and congenital abnormalities. *The Lancet* **2**: 1358.

17) Warkany, J (1988) Why I doubted that thalidomide was the cause of the epidemic of limb defects of 1959 to 1961. *Teratology* **38** 217-19.

18) Lenz, W (1965) Epidemiology of congenital malformations. *Ann. NY Acad. Sci.* **123** 228-36.

19) Somers, G F (1963) The foetal toxicity of thalidomide. *Proc. European Soc. Study Drug Toxicity* **1** 49.

20) King, C T G and Kendrick, F J (1962) Teratogenic effects of thalidomide in the Sprague Dawley rat. *The Lancet* **2** 1116.

21) McColl, J D, Globus, M and Robinson, S (1965) Effect of some therapeutic agents on the developing rat fetus. *Toxicol. appl. Pharmacol.* **7** 409-17.

22) Christie, G A (1962) Thalidomide and congenital abnormalities. *The Lancet* **2** 249.

23) Fabro, S, Smith, R L and Williams, R T (1967) Toxicity and teratogenicity of optical isomers of thalidomide. *Nature* **215** 296.

24) Shah, R R, Midgeley, J M and Branch, S K (1998) Stereochemical origin of some clinically significant drug safety concerns: lessons for future drug development. *Adverse Drug React. Toxicol Rev.* **17** 145-90.

25) Schumacher, H, Smith, R L and Williams, R T (1965) The metabolism of thalidomide: The spontaneous hydrolysis of thalidomide in solution. *Brit. J. Pharmacol.* **25** 324-27.

26) Thalidomide Patent 1957. *British Patent* 768,821.

27) Fox, R R, Sawin, P B, Crary, D D and Wuest, H M (1966) Intravenous injection of thalidomide in pregnant rabbits. *Science* **153** 310.

28) Schumacher, H, Blake, D and Gillette, J (1966) Thalidomide solutions. *Science* **154** 1362.

29) Wuest, H M and Fox, R R (1966) Thalidomide solutions. *Science* **154** 1362.

30) Runner, M N (1967) Comparative pharmacology in relation to teratogenesis. *Fed. Proc.* **26** 1131-36.

31) Bazzoli, A S, Manson, J, Scott, W J and Wilson, J G (1977) The effects of thalidomide on the generating forelimb of the newt. *J. Embryol. Exp. Morphol.* **41** 125-35.

32) Shah, R R (2001) Thalidomide, drug safety and early drug regulation in the U.K. *Adv. Drug React. Toxicol. Rev.* **20** 199-255.

33) Association of the British Pharmaceutical Industry (1964) First Report of the Expert Committee on Drug Toxicity together with further Recommendations on Toxicity Evaluation.

34) 1992. Press advertisement in the U.K. by the Antivivisection Agency.

35) Advertising Standards Authority Report, Ref. B92-02904.

36) Greek, C R and Greek, J S (2000) *Sacred Cows and Golden Geese.* New York: Continuum.

19. Misleading Research or Misleading Statistics: Animal Experiments and Cancer Research

Scientists supported by the Cancer Research Campaign have prepared a vaccine which it is hoped will protect against infection with Epstein-Barr virus (EBV). Apart from causing glandular fever EBV is believed to be one causative factor for certain cancers. There is firm evidence for the involvement of this virus in Burkitt's lymphoma and in cancer of the throat and nasopharynx, and evidence for the suggested link between EBV and Hodgkin's disease is becoming more conclusive.

Progress has recently been made in the search for a vaccine against the Epstein-Barr virus. A new vaccine has undergone Phase I clinical trials in China, where there is a high incidence of nasopharyngeal carcinoma caused by the Epstein-Barr virus (21). Progress to Phase III trials of this vaccine has been recommended by a recent meeting of cancer experts (22).

Should the vaccine prove successful, its widespread use will ultimately prevent approximately 80,000 deaths per year world-wide.

To the scientist involved in research into the prevention and cure of neoplastic disease this news will be viewed as another significant step in the steady progress made over the last 50 years in reducing mortality from cancer.

Those devoted to attacking the scientific credibility of researchers who use animals, however, look to cancer research to provide evidence to support their campaign to achieve the abolition of animal experiments.

In a recent article (1) it is claimed that despite the continued use of animals there is still an "inexorable rise in cancer mortality." The claim is allegedly

http://dx.doi.org/10.11647/OBP.0055.19

supported by selected examples of mortality figures for various cancers for
1981-85 compared to 1971-75, with the percentage change listed.

Such carefully chosen statistics provide limited information to the serious
investigator. If the change in incidence is also included one can see that the
increase in mortality is small in comparison with the increase in incidence
(Fig. 19.1). The apparent increase in incidence is undoubtedly due to a
general increase in longevity and also because the percentage of actual cancer
patients surviving longer than 5 years has increased steadily in England and
Wales since 1960. The more recent statistics (1988) for the USA indicate that
this trend is being maintained.

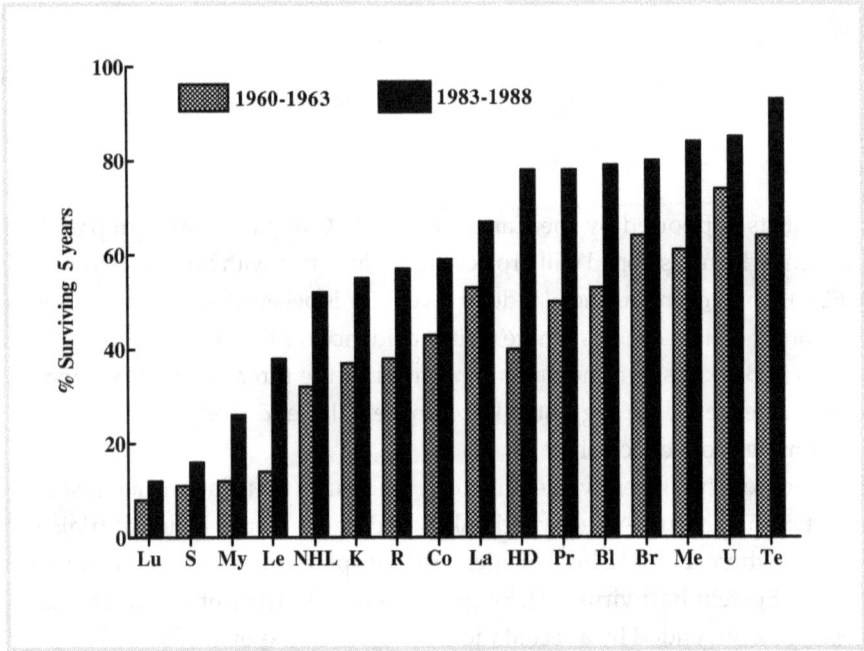

Fig. 19.1 Trends in cancer survival in the USA (male and female white), 1960-1963 and
1983-1988. Lu: lung; S: stomach; My: myeloma; Le: leukaemias; NHL: non-Hodgkin's
lymphoma; K: kidney; R: rectum; Co: colon; La: larynx; HD: Hodgkin's disease; Pr:
prostate; Bl: bladder; Br: breast; ME: melanoma; U: uterus; Te: testis.

If mortalities from cancer for different age groups are examined, changes
over the last 30 years show an encouraging trend. In the age group 0-19
years mortality from cancer has dropped to under half that in 1953, in
those 20-44 to 65% and in those 44-64 to 80%. Only in those aged over 65
has the mortality risen, this because of the increased longevity mentioned

above. Earlier diagnosis may be a factor in the increased survival time, but undoubtedly improved treatment is significant (Fig. 19.2).

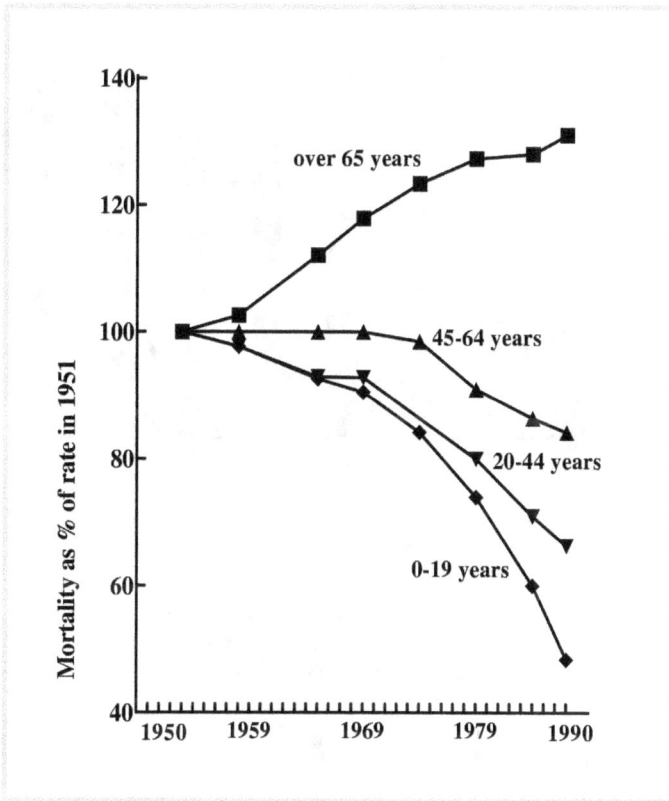

Fig. 19.2 Trends in cancer mortality in England and Wales (males), 1950-1990.

In fact, the prognosis for some cancers has improved markedly. 95% of patients with disseminated cancer of the testis are now cured,[1] 40-50% of patients with acute non-lymphocytic or chronic myelogenous leukaemia are also curable (2). Fortunately, the most striking progress has occurred in the treatment of childhood cancers, where 5 year survival rates have shown a striking increase over the past 30 years, with high cure rates for the childhood leukaemias and even for solid tumours (Fig. 19.3). It is perhaps significant that these statistics were not chosen for inclusion in the report referred to (1).

---

1   "It is certainly fortunate that the platinum drugs were discovered when they were, or it (cancer of the testis) would by now be a major cause of death in young men." Sir Richard Doll (1990) Are we winning the war against cancer? *Eur J Cancer* **76** 500-508.

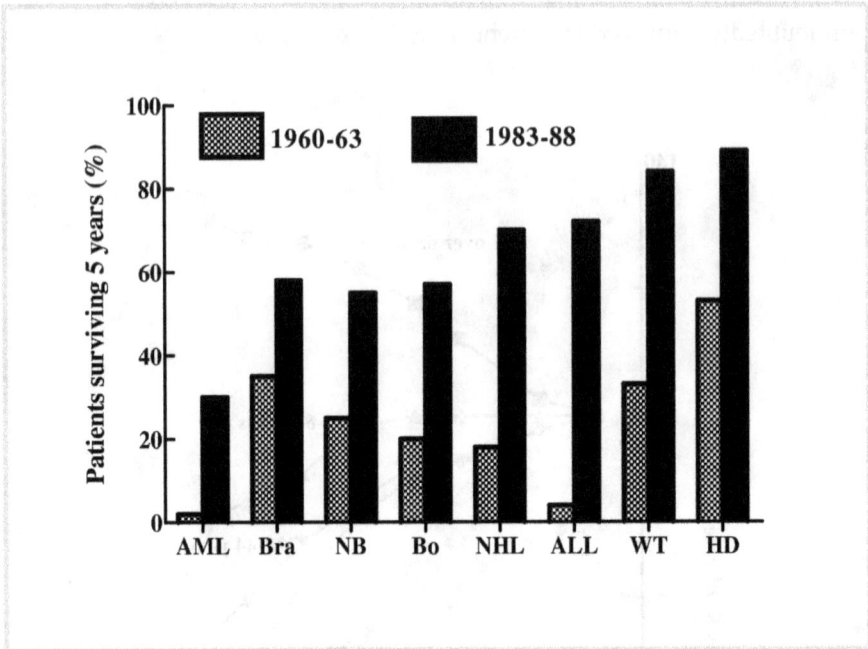

Fig. 19.3   Trends in survival of children under 15 in the USA, 1960-1963 and 1983-1988. AML: Acute myeloid leukaemia; Bra: brain; NB: neuroblastoma; Bo: bone; NHL: non-Hodgkin's lymphoma; ALL: acute lymphocytic leukaemia; WT: Wilm's tumour; HD: Hodgkin's disease.

Chemotherapy

Unquestionably, the great improvements in cure rate for childhood cancer and increased life expectancy for cancer patients in general is due to the development of chemotherapy with antineoplastic agents.

Before 1940 there were no anticancer drugs. The first (1941) edition of a standard textbook on the pharmacological basis of therapeutics does not even mention cancer in the index. The eighth edition (1990) devotes 61 pages to the discussion of some 40-50 antineoplastic drugs (3).

The starting point of this dramatic change in cancer treatment was the investigation of the biological and chemical actions of the nitrogen mustards by Gilman and Philips (4). Although not published until 1946, this work was actually initiated prior to World War II due to the possible use of these vesicants in chemical warfare. For reasons of security publication was delayed.

The striking toxic action of nitrogen mustards on lymphoid tissue prompted experiments upon the effects of these chemicals on transplanted lymphosarcoma in mice (5). The suppression of tumour growth observed in this study was responsible for the first clinical investigation of a medicine to combat cancer (6).

Numerous other anticancer drugs have now been produced. Aminopterin, shown to be effective in treating various experimental neoplasms (7), actinomycin D, effective against five experimental tumours (8) and vincristine, isolated from the periwinkle (*Vinca rosa*). This drug was initially shown to produce bone marrow depression in animals and hence was used in an experimental leukaemia model where it was shown to be curative (9).

As knowledge of the mode of action of anticancer drugs unfolded so did the production of analogues with increased potential, either because of greater activity or diminished toxicity. This necessitated the investigation of the effectiveness of potential methods to screen compounds for activity. This was undertaken as a co-operative venture involving many national centres. Numerous *in vitro* systems were examined for the investigation of potential anti-tumour activity, including various mammalian cells in culture, bacteria, fungi and viruses (10). However the results indicated that no *in vitro* method could replace a whole animal tumour model (some drugs, cyclophosphamide for example, were only active *in vivo* after conversion in the liver to an active form). Furthermore, the use of no single animal tumour model could with certainty discover all the potentially useful drugs. Thus three mouse tumour models were selected for an initial screen; leukaemia L1210 (for its good predictive value for clinical activity), sarcoma 180 and adenocarcinoma 755 (these for their cytological similarity to human cancers) (10).

As more compounds were produced, tested and forwarded for clinical assessment, feedback from oncologists as to clinical efficacy enabled the experimental test systems to be reassessed and thus various other animal tumour sytems were found useful, such as the P388 mouse leukaemia, mouse B16 melanotic melanoma and the mouse Lewis lung carcinoma. The informative review by Johnson and Goldin (10) contains a table of 34 chemicals established as active against one or more human cancers. Most were effective in prolonging the life of mice with L1210 and P338 leukaemia, the majority were also active against B16 melanoma. Few clinically effective drugs failed to show an activity against at least one of the established animal tumour models.

It is of interest that one critic of the contribution of animal research towards the treatment of cancer (1) surprisingly cites the above paper as evidence of the futility of animal models, since *"estrogen (sic) is effective against some cancers in women but, like prednisone fails to work in animal experiments."* To use these two drugs as evidence to diminish the value of experimental tumour systems, and to ignore the concordance of response of these experimental tumours and human cancers to the other drugs listed indicates remarkable prejudice, together with a superficial knowledge of cancer chemotherapy. Certainly, both prednisone and sex hormones were listed as inactive against the four experimental tumours examined. Prednisone and other corticosteroids seldom exert benefit in adult leukaemias and only produce cures in childhood leukaemias if given in combination with other antineoplastic agents. Oestrogen is only used for cancer of the breast (no experimental mammary cancer model was used) and then only in carefully selected patients. In fact oestrogen antagonists such as tamoxifen are more often used. (Oestrogens have of course been established as cancer causing when administered under some conditions, an action predicted by studies in the mouse by Lacassagne (11) and subsequently confirmed in other animal species).

Treatment Regimens

Animal models were not only of use for the generation of novel anticancer drugs, but were also crucial for the establishment of the principles that underpin modern cancer chemotherapy.

Using only the L1210 mouse leukaemia model, Skipper and co-workers (12) demonstrated that; 1) since a single malignant cell can divide and eventually form enough cells to kill the host, it is essential to destroy every such cell. 2) The immune system plays little or no part in the therapy of malignant disease, and 3) the destruction of cancer cells by cytotoxic drugs follows first order kinetics, i.e. a given dose of drug will kill a fixed proportion of sensitive cells regardless of the total size of the malignancy.

The consequence of these experimental studies has been to ensure total removal of malignant cells originally, by continuance of therapy after apparent remission, and later by the use of several drugs concurrently or in a logical sequence.

These studies emphasised the importance of the influence of tumour cell numbers at the start of therapy as an indicator of a favourable outcome (methotrexate, for example, was only curative in mice when treatment was started shortly after inoculation of a small number of cells). This observation did much to encourage research into methods of early diagnosis of malignant disease, since treatment at an asymptomatic stage increases the probability of a cure.

The Alternatives?

The alternative to animal experiments, assert the abolitionists, is epidemiology. To support this proposal a paper by the eminent epidemiologist Burkitt has been cited (13), in which it is argued that a "shift in emphasis towards prevention" is required. Few would dream of disagreeing that epidemiology, and ultimately prevention, is of paramount importance in the field of cancer research and indeed of most diseases. The discussion paper by Temple and Burkitt does not however support the abandonment of animal experiments. It is a plea for "simple" as against "complex" research and specifically states:

> it (simple research) should use several types of investigation in parallel: (1) population comparisons, (2) prospective and case-control studies, (3) controlled clinical trials, (4) *analogous studies on animals,* and (5) envisaging a plausible mechanism.

It is surprising that Sharpe, in support of his condemnation of the past and future contribution of animal experimentation to research into cancer (1), should quote so extensively from a paper that specifically recommends animal experiments.

Reducing the Toxicity of Anticancer Therapy

All cancer chemotherapy is accompanied by unpleasant effects, since the drugs used are all cytotoxic, the selectivity against the cancer cells being governed by the accelerated rate of division of these cells. Research using animals has however, provided adjunctive therapy that has greatly eased the suffering of the patient.

One of the most discomforting symptoms accompanying anticancer chemotherapy or radiotherapy is nausea and vomiting. This can be combated with dramatic effectiveness with the newly developed 5-HT3 receptor antagonists. Two of these drugs, ondansetron and granisetron, are now widely used in cancer clinics to suppress completely the nausea and vomiting that accompanies treatment. The potential of these drugs was established by the demonstration that they could potently inhibit retching and vomiting induced in ferrets by cisplatin (14).

Since new blood cells are constantly being formed from rapidly dividing stem cells in the bone marrow, this organ is inevitably affected by anticancer therapy. Supportive therapy can help to alleviate this problem, for example prevention of anaemia can be achieved by the administration of factors, such as erythropoietin, that promote the formation of red blood cells. This has only been made possible by the elucidation of the circulating factors responsible for the maturation of red blood cells, starting with the significant experiments on rabbits by Carnot and Deflandre (15).

The Future

Though it is clearly justified to emphasise the progress that has been made in the treatment of cancer, it must be admitted that slow growing tumours, such as those in the lung and colon, are generally difficult to treat and are amongst the biggest killers, often because of the generation of metastases. The elucidation of the processes by which metastases develop can only be achieved by the study of tumour development and spread in laboratory animals.

A promising approach to the possibility of suppression of metastases has emerged from the observation by Folkman (16) that the antibiotic fumagillin inhibits the growth of the cells that line the inner surface of blood vessels, the endothelial cells. It is the endothelial cells that initiate the growth of new blood vessels, and tumours cannot grow above a few millimetres in size unless they can form blood vessels. A relatively non-toxic derivative of fumagillin has been shown to reduce substantially the number of metastases in mice, presumably by the inhibition of the growth of blood vessels.

Similarly one can anticipate that monoclonal antibodies (originally generated from tumour antigens) may contribute to diagnosis, imaging of tumours and to therapy, perhaps by being made to deliver a toxin or destructive radioisotope selectively to the tumour.

In some respects cancer therapy today is analogous to bacterial chemotherapy in the early 1930s. Decades of research looking for compounds that would kill the bacterial cell and leave intact the surrounding, rather similar, host tissue had produced somewhat hazardous treatments for a few conditions. But death and morbidity rates for common infections were high. Over a span of a mere seven years or so the sulphonamides and then the antibiotics had rendered infectious disease a relatively minor medical problem.

Gene therapy, the biological response modifiers and maybe a vaccine against tumour antigens (17) (in conjunction with suitable adjuvant therapy) may provide the turning point that will make the successful treatment of neoplasms routine medicine.

In recent years, the development of vaccines to prevent or treat some cancers has progressed significantly. The FDA has approved two vaccines to prevent cancer. One is a vaccine against the hepatitis B virus which can cause liver cancer (18) and the other is a vaccine against the papillomavirus, which is responsible for the majority of cervical cancer cases (19). Also, in 2010, the FDA approved the first cancer treatment vaccine for use in a particular group of men with metastatic prostate cancer. This vaccine, sipuleucel-T, is designed to stimulate an immune response to prostatic acid phosphatase, an antigen found on most prostate cancer cells (20).

Vaccines for the treatment of many forms of cancer, such as cancers of the bladder, kidney and lung, are the subject of current extensive studies.

An earlier version of this chapter was published as: Misleading research or misleading statistics – animal experiments and cancer research. *RDS News* April 1993 6-9.

References

1) Sharpe R (1991) The War Against Cancer. *Outrage*. No 74 Jun/Jul.

2) Chabner B, Rothenberg M (1991) Medical oncology in the 1990s. *The Lancet* **338**, 576-77.

3) Goodman L, Gilman A (1990) *The Pharmacological Basis of Therapeutics*. 8th Edition.

4) Gilman A, Philips F (1946) The biological actions and therapeutic applications of the beta-chloroethylamines and sulphides. *Science* **103** 409-15.

5) Goodman L, Gilman A & Daugherty T (1942) unpublished observations, referred to in Goodman L et al (1946). *JAMA* **132** 126-32.

6) Gilman A (1963) The initial clinical trial of nitrogen mustard. *Am J Surg* **105** 574-78.

7) Sugiura K, Moore A, Stock C (1949) The effect of aminopterin on the growth of carcinoma, sarcoma and melanoma in animals. *Cancer* **2** 491-502.

8) Sugiura K (1960) The effect of actinomycin D on a spectrum of tumors. *Ann NY Acad Sci* **89** 368-372.

9) Johnson I, Armstrong J, Gorman M and Burnett J (1963) The Vinca alkaloids: a new class of oncolytic agents. *Cancer Res* **23** 1390-1427.

10) Johnson R, Goldin A (1975) The clinical impact of screening and other experimental tumor studies. *Cancer Treatment Reviews* **2** 1-31.

11) Lacassagne A (1936) Tumeurs malignes appareus au cours d'un traitement hormonal combine chez de souris appartenant a des lignees refractaire au cancer spontane. *C R Soc Biol (Paris)* **121** 607-09.

12) Skipper H, Schabel F (1973) Quantitative and cytokinetic studies in experimental tumor models, in *Cancer Medicine* eds Holland J & Frei E Lea & Febiger pp 629-50.

13) Temple N, Burkitt D (1991) The war on cancer – failure of therapy and research: discussion paper. *J Roy Soc Med* **84** 95-98.

14) Bunce K. Tyers M. & Beranek P. (1991) Clinical evaluation of 5HT3 receptor antagonists as anti-emetics. *TIPS* **12** 46-48.

15) Carnot P, Deflandre C (1906) Sur l'activite hemopoietique de serum au cours de la regeneration du sang. *CR Acad Sci (III)* **143** 384-86.

16) (1991) Exploiting angiogenesis. *The Lancet* **337** 208-09.

17) Pullen L C (2011) Epstein-Barr virus vaccine may soon enter Phase 3 Trial. *Medscape*. Nov 07, 2011, www.medscape.com.

18) Barry M, Cooper C (2007) Review of hepatitis B surface antigen-1018 ISS adjuvant-containing vaccine; safety and efficacy. *Expert Opin Biol. Ther.* **7**, 1731-37.

19) Tay EH, Garland S, Tang G et al. (2008) Clinical trial experience with prophylactic HPV 6/11/16/18 VLP vaccine in young women from the asia-pacific region. *Int. J.Gynaecol. Obstet.* **102** 275-83.

20) Kantoff P W, Higano C S, Shore N D et al. (2010) Sipuleucel-T immunotherapy for castration resistant prostate cancer. *N Engl J Med* **363** 411-22.

21) Hui E P, Taylor G S, Hui J et al. (2012) Phase I trial of recombinant modified *vaccinia ankara* encoding Epstein-Barr viral tumor antigens in nasopharyngeal carcinoma patients. *Cancer Res* **73** 1676-88.

22) Fauci A S, Varmus H, Nabel G and Cohen J (2011) Epstein-Barr virus vaccine may soon enter Phase III trial. *Sci Transl Med* **3** 107fs7 (abstract).

Index

This book need not end here...

At Open Book Publishers, we are changing the nature of the traditional academic book. The title you have just read will not be left on a library shelf, but will be accessed online by hundreds of readers each month across the globe. We make all our books free to read online so that students, researchers and members of the public who can't afford a printed edition can still have access to the same ideas as you.

Our digital publishing model also allows us to produce online supplementary material, including extra chapters, reviews, links and other digital resources. Find *Animals and Medicine* on our website to access its online extras. Please check this page regularly for ongoing updates, and join the conversation by leaving your own comments:

http://www.openbookpublishers.com/isbn/9781783741175

If you enjoyed this book, and feel that research like this should be available to all readers, regardless of their income, please think about donating to us. Our company is run entirely by academics, and our publishing decisions are based on intellectual merit and public value rather than on commercial viability. We do not operate for profit and all donations, as with all other revenue we generate, will be used to finance new Open Access publications.

For further information about what we do, how to donate to OBP, additional digital material related to our titles or to order our books, please visit our website: http://www.openbookpublishers.com

OpenBook
Publishers
Knowledge is for sharing

www.ingramcontent.com/pod-product-compliance
Lightning Source LLC
Chambersburg PA
CBHW061156220326
41599CB00025B/4496